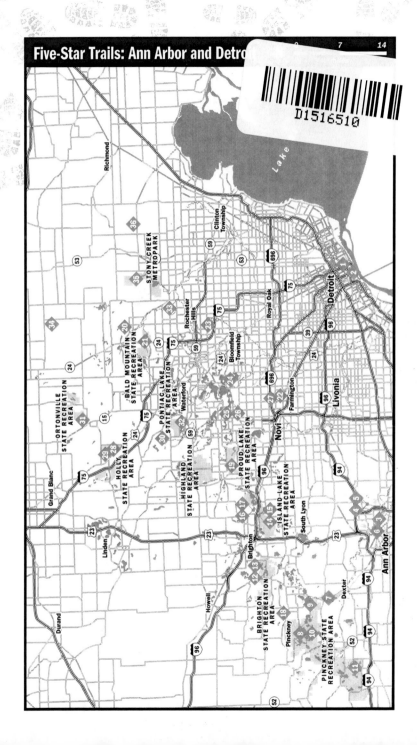

Map Legend

Trailhead	North Indicator	Path Direction	Off map or pinpoint	Capital, Cities and towns

Interstate highways	U.S. highways	State roads	Other roads	Unpaved roads

Featured trail	Alternate trail	Boardwalk or stairs	Powerline	Railroads

River or stream	Water body	Marsh	Preserve or other public land

Amphitheater	Fishing	Phone access
Barn	Food service	Playground
Beach access	Garden	Ranger station
Bench	Gate	Restrooms
Bicycle trail	General Point of Interest	RV campground
Boardwalk	Golf course	RV sanitation dump
Boat launch	Hiking trail	Scenic viewpoint
Bridge	Hospital	Shelter
Campfire area	Information	Shooting range
Campground	Lookout tower	Stable
Canoe access	Marina	Swimming
Cemetery	Overlook	Tennis court
Church	Parking	Tunnel
Dam	Pavilion	Viewing area
Equestrian trail	Peak	Water access
First aid	Picnic	

Overview Map Key

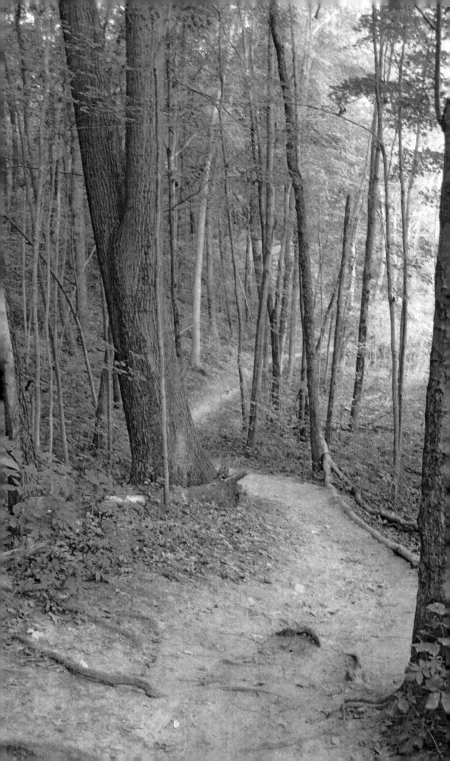

Five-Star
Trails

Ann Arbor
and Detroit

Your Guide to the Area's Most Beautiful Hikes

Greg Tasker

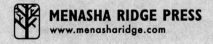

MENASHA RIDGE PRESS
www.menasharidge.com

Five-Star Trails: Ann Arbor & Detroit
Your Guide to the Area's Most Beautiful Hikes

Copyright © 2011 by Greg Tasker
All rights reserved
Published by Menasha Ridge Press
Distributed by Publishers Group West
Printed in the United States of America
First edition, first printing

Cover design by Scott McGrew
Cover photographs by Greg Tasker
Frontispiece: Along the Crooked Lake Trail (see page 63)
Text design by Annie Long
Author photograph by Victoria Valan
Interior photographs by Greg Tasker and Roni Leibovitch (page 155)
Cartography and elevation profiles by Scott McGrew
Indexing by Rich Carlson

Library of Congress Cataloging-in-Publication Data

Tasker, Greg.
 Five-star trails, Ann Arbor and Detroit: your guide to the area's most beautiful
hikes/Greg Tasker. —1st ed.
   p. cm.
 Summary: "Each hike features an individual trail map, elevation profile, and at-a-
glance information, helping readers quickly find the perfect trip. Sized to fit in a
pocket, the book's detailed trail descriptions will help readers find their way on and off
the trail. Driving directions and GPS trailhead coordinates will help with navigating
the myriad of unnamed roads. The trails covered range from those best suited to the
novice, families, experienced hikers, or backpackers."—Provided by publisher.
 ISBN-13: 978-0-89732-952-1 (pbk.)
 ISBN-10: 0-89732-952-X ()
 1. Hiking—Michigan—Ann Arbor—Guidebooks. 2. Hiking—Michigan—Detroit—
Guidebooks. 3. Trails—Michigan—Ann Arbor—Guidebooks. 4. Trails—Michigan—
Detroit—Guidebooks. 5. Michigan—Guidebooks. I. Title.
 GV199.42.M5T37 2011
 917.743—dc22
                        2011015832

Menasha Ridge Press
P.O. Box 43673
Birmingham, AL 35243
menasharidgepress.com

Contents

Dedication

*To my grandmother Delia Marsh and my late grandfather
Ronald LaForge, who led memorable treks into the
northern Michigan woods and planted the seeds for
a lifelong affinity for hiking and nature.*

Acknowledgments

I would like to thank the Sierra Club for helping me gain a sense of the variety and abundance of trails in southeast Michigan. Its comprehensive list of day-hiking areas around Detroit was an invaluable guide. Club leaders' suggestions included such gems as the Lloyd A. Stage Nature Center in Troy and the Orchard Lake Nature Sanctuary—woodsy escapes in the middle of suburbia. Both are included in this book.

Recommendations for trails also came from other sources, including members of the Michigan Adventurers Club; we share enthusiasm for many of the same hikes in metro Detroit and Ann Arbor. The staff at state recreation areas and metroparks also were helpful in making suggestions and providing details on fauna, foliage, and history.

One of my constant companions on the trail during three springs and falls of hiking was my mom. Thanks for your eagerness to explore with me, and for your company. Hiking with my daughters, Courtney and Chelsea, made for memorable autumn outings.

And to a host of friends—John, Roni, Molly, Kevin, Cindy, Christopher, Peter, William, Michelle, Billy, and Kellie—thanks for coming along and for your interest in the book.

And lastly, to the staff at Menasha Ridge Press. Scott McGrew, thanks for dealing with my maps. And to my editors: Molly Merkle, I appreciate your patience; and Susan Haynes, thanks for helping me to narrow the book's focus, to get organized, and to get back on track.

Preface

You *can* hike in metropolitan Detroit.

That comes as a surprise to most people.

It came as a surprise to me.

That's because my first hike in the region—a few years ago—was a disaster. I no sooner stepped on a trail at a state recreation area than I was run over by an endless parade of mountain bikers. My guidebook never mentioned that bikers used the trail. And the attendant at the park entrance gave no warning either, even though I asked several questions about the trail.

For a long time I thought hiking in metropolitan Detroit was a lost cause, but in researching this book, I learned that the region is rife with trails. Hiking is an outdoor pursuit that gets little attention, despite an abundance of trails at state recreation areas, metroparks, county parks, and nature centers. While these trails lack vistas as rewards for a day's hike, they are no less scenic as they pass through hardwood forests, wetlands, and prairies and around lakes. Hike one in late September or early October with oaks and maples ablaze with color, and you'd be hard-pressed to find a more captivating landscape anywhere.

What's more, the region is home to one of the most extensive network of rail-trails, abandoned rail lines turned into recreational paths, in the country. Two of the most popular, Paint Creek Trail and the West Bloomfield Trail, are featured in this book. Both are gentle trails that pass through varied terrain near picturesque communities. The trails, too, provide glimpses of nature even as they traverse urban areas. They also connect to other rail-trails, uniting communities from one end of Oakland County to the other. And you will have to share these trails with bikers, runners, and inline skaters.

If a hike in the city is more to your liking, you won't do better than the Detroit RiverWalk and the Dequindre Cut Greenway. The RiverWalk runs along the Detroit River from Joe Louis Arena to William G. Milliken State Park and Harbor, east of the Renaissance

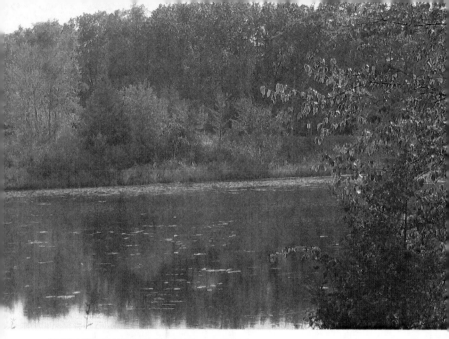

STONY CREEK METROPARK, EAST LAKE TRAILS

Center in downtown Detroit. The pathway offers great views of the river and Windsor and Detroit landmarks. It ends at a beautiful state park, Michigan's only urban state park. The RiverWalk is connected to another urban trail, the Dequindre Cut Greenway, which juts north along an old commuter rail line from Rivertown to Eastern Market. The market is an ideal ending or beginning on Saturdays when the market is abuzz with vendors selling vegetables, fruits, canned and baked goods, flowers, and meats. Just over a mile long, the trail runs mostly below street level, and its cement walls have become canvases for graffiti artists.

You don't even have to leave the suburbs to escape into the woods. The West Bloomfield Nature Preserve, Orchard Lake Nature Sanctuary, and the Lloyd A. Stage Nature Center in Troy are oases amid urban sprawl. The Orchard Lake Nature Sanctuary, just down the road from the West Bloomfield Woods Nature Preserve, is home to one of the last stands of old-growth forest in the metropolitan region. Its trails crisscross thick woods between two lakes in northern Oakland County.

If those recreation areas were not enough, the region also boasts well-known metroparks. While the parks draw tens of thousands for boating, swimming, golf, and other activities, they're also home to some wonderful trails. The metropark trails are among the best-maintained and well-marked trails in the region. They pass through second-growth woodlands and prairies and around rivers and lakes. Many include interpretive signs that explain the foliage, fauna, and wildlife. Many of them touch upon the region's past, with restored mills and farms as focal points of the expansive parks.

Even more surprising are the state recreation areas located around the fringes of the region. These expansive parks cover some of the most rugged terrain in southeast Michigan and, in some cases, offer hikers the experience of Up North. The parks are thick with woods, rolling terrain, deep ravines, lakes, and wetlands. Pinckney State Recreation Area best exemplifies the sense of northern Michigan backcountry, but you will share some of the trails with bikers. Neighboring state recreation areas—Island Lake, Brighton, and Proud Lake—come close to replicating a more primitive landscape.

And there are many more, smaller trails out there. But this book focuses on the best the region has to offer. So pick a trail. and get out and enjoy the natural beauty of southeast Michigan.

Recommended Hikes

Best for Scenery

Best for Wildlife

Best for Seclusion

Best for Kids

Best for Wildflowers

Best for Swimming

Best for Picnics

Best for Fall Colors

Best for Cross-country Skiing

Introduction

About This Book

While southeast Michigan might not spring immediately to mind as hiking country, the region's diverse landscape, including woodlands, wetlands, lakes, rivers, prairies—and even hills—makes it ideal for a variety of enjoyable day hikes.

With the exception of the urban trails in Detroit and the rail-trails in the suburbs, the trails featured in this book all pass through notable woodlands. The dominant forests are hardwoods, composed of oak, maple, beech, and hickory. Except for a pocket or two, old-growth forests are long gone from the region, victims of 19th- and 20th-century settlement, farming, and urban expansion. Fortunately, one of the trails included here—at Orchard Lake Nature Sanctuary—winds through one of the region's last vestiges of old-growth forests. It's an impressive site, one not to be missed. Second-growth forests have reclaimed some of the land, and the trails at state recreation areas, metroparks, and nature centers pass through formidable woodlands, home to a variety of wildlife and songbirds.

While none of the trails included here touch upon the region's great lakes—that is, Erie and St. Clair—many of them touch the shorelines of some of the countless inland lakes that dot southeast Michigan. Some trails, such as Losee Lake, Silver Lake, and Crooked Lake, are named after them. Trails also crisscross and wind along some of the region's most prominent rivers—Detroit, Huron, and Clinton and their tributaries. It's a rare trail that doesn't pass by some form of water. Wetlands, too, abound, and you won't hike too far without passing or cutting through marshlands or swamps. Count on boardwalks to help guide you through expansive or thick wetlands.

You'll even find hills in southeast Michigan, especially in the state recreation areas on the fringes of the metropolitan region. You'll find more rugged terrain in Pinckney, Island Lake, and Brighton state recreation areas on the west side, and in Bald Mountain and Holly state recreation areas in northern Oakland County. Some hills are more formidable than others, but the elevations never rise more than a couple hundred feet from the trailhead.

One of the lesser-known topographical features of southeastern Michigan is the prairie. Once commonplace before settlement and farming, prairies—remnants or reconstructed—can be found along several trails, including the Marilyn Bland Prairie Trail at Matthaei Botanical Gardens in Ann Arbor. But you'll also find prairies at the Nichols Arboretum in Ann Arbor, Seven Ponds Nature Center, and along the Paint Creek Trail in northern Oakland County. The reconstructed prairie at Seven Ponds may be the most inviting; trails crisscross tall grasses, and a strategically placed tower offers a sweeping view of the landscape.

Lastly, when most people think of southeastern Michigan, cities spring to mind. Two trails included here are strictly urban. The Dequindre Cut Greenway runs along an old commuter rail line into downtown Detroit, ending just beyond the riverfront. Along the riverfront, the Detroit RiverWalk follows the Detroit River from Joe Louis Arena to a small urban state park at its eastern end. This promenade offers stunning views of the river as well as the Detroit and Windsor skylines.

How to Use This Guidebook

The following information walks you through this guidebook's organization to make it easy and convenient for you to plan great hikes.

Overview Map, Map Key, & Map Legend

The overview map on the inside front cover depicts the location of the primary trailhead for all 36 hikes in this book. The numbers shown on the overview map pair with the map key on the first page. Each hike's number remains with that hike throughout the book. Thus, if you spot an appealing hiking area on the overview map, you can flip through the book and find those hikes easily by their numbers at the top of each profile page.

Trail Maps

In addition to the overview map, a detailed map of each hike's route appears with its profile. On this map, symbols indicate the trailhead, the complete route, significant features, facilities, and topographic landmarks such as creeks, overlooks, and peaks. A legend identifying the map symbols used throughout the book appears on the inside back cover.

To produce the highly accurate maps in this book, I used a handheld GPS unit to gather data while hiking each route, and then sent that data to the publisher's expert cartographers. Your GPS is not really a substitute for sound, sensible navigation according to conditions on the ground. Most of the trails in this book are actually quite easy to follow, so where they differ from our imaginary lines, stay on the trail.

Further, despite the high quality of the maps in this guidebook, the publisher and I strongly recommend that you always carry an additional map, such as the ones noted in each entry's "Maps" listing.

Elevation Profile (diagram)

For trails with significant elevation changes, the hike description will include this graphic profile. Entries for fairly flat routes, such as a lake loop, will not display an elevation profile graph.

Also, each entry will list the elevation at the hike trailhead, and it will list the elevation peak if there is any notable elevation change for that trail. Otherwise, the entry will simply indicate the trailhead elevation.

For hike descriptions where the elevation profile is included, this diagram represents the rises and falls of the trail as viewed from the side, over the complete distance (in miles) of that trail. On the diagram's vertical axis, or height scale, the number of feet indicated between each tick mark lets you visualize the climb. To avoid making flat hikes look steep and steep hikes appear flat, varying height scales provide an accurate image of each hike's climbing difficulty. For example, one hike's scale might rise to 1,008 feet, while another reaches 1,130 feet.

The Hike Profile

This book contains a concise and informative narrative of each hike from beginning to end. The text will get you from a well-known road or highway to the trailhead, to the twists and turns of the hike route, back to the trailhead, and to notable nearby attractions, if there are any. Each profile opens with the route's star ratings, GPS trailhead coordinates, and other key information. Below is an explanation of the introductory elements that give you a snapshot of each of this book's 36 routes.

STAR RATINGS

Five-Star Trails is the Menasha Ridge Press series title of guidebooks geared to specific cities across the United States, such as this one for Ann Arbor and Detroit. Following is the explanation for the rating system of one to five stars in each of the five categories.

FOR SCENERY:

★ ★ ★ ★ ★   Unique, picturesque panoramas

★ ★ ★ ★   Diverse vistas

★ ★ ★   Pleasant views

★ ★   Unchanging landscape

★   Not selected for scenery

FOR TRAIL CONDITION:

★ ★ ★ ★ ★   Consistently well maintained

★ ★ ★ ★   Stable, with no surprises

★ ★ ★   Average terrain to negotiate

★ ★   Inconsistent, with good and poor areas

★   Rocky, overgrown, or often muddy

FOR CHILDREN:

★ ★ ★ ★ ★   Babes in strollers are welcome

★ ★ ★ ★   Fun for anyone past the toddler stage

★ ★ ★   Good for young hikers with proven stamina

★ ★   Not enjoyable for children

★   Not advisable for children

FOR DIFFICULTY:

★ ★ ★ ★ ★   Grueling

★ ★ ★ ★   Strenuous

★ ★ ★   Moderate (won't beat you up—but you'll know you've been hiking)

★ ★   Easy with patches of moderate

★   Good for a relaxing stroll

FOR SOLITUDE:

★ ★ ★ ★ ★   Positively tranquil

★ ★ ★ ★   Spurts of isolation

★ ★ ★   Moderately secluded

★ ★   Crowded on weekends and holidays

★   Steady stream of individuals and/or groups

GPS Trailhead Coordinates

As noted in "Trail Maps" previously, I used a handheld GPS unit to obtain geographic data and sent the information to the publisher's cartographers. In the opener for each hike profile, I have provided the intersection of the latitude (north) and longitude (west) coordinates to orient you at the trailhead. In some cases, you can drive within viewing distance of a trailhead. Other hikes require a short walk to reach the trailhead from a parking area. Either way, the trailhead coordinates are given from the trail's actual head—its point of origin.

You will also note that this guidebook uses the degree–decimal minute format for presenting the latitude and longitude GPS coordinates.

The latitude and longitude grid system is likely quite familiar to you, but here is a refresher, pertinent to visualizing the GPS coordinates. Imaginary lines of latitude—called parallels and approximately 69 miles apart from each other—run horizontally around the globe. Each parallel is indicated by degrees from the equator (established to be 0°) up to 90°N at the North Pole and down to 90°S at the South Pole.

Imaginary lines of longitude—called meridians—run perpendicular to latitude lines. Longitude lines are likewise indicated by degrees starting from 0° at the Prime Meridian in Greenwich, England, and they continue to the east and west until they meet 180° later at the International Date Line in the Pacific Ocean. At the equator, longitude lines also are approximately 69 miles apart, but that distance narrows as the meridians converge toward the North and South poles.

To convert GPS coordinates given in degrees, minutes, and seconds to the format shown above in degrees–decimal minutes, the seconds are divided by 60. For more information on GPS technology, visit **usgs.gov.**

DISTANCE & CONFIGURATION

The distance shown is for the hike from start to finish, as recorded with the GPS unit. There may be options to shorten or extend the hike, but the mileage corresponds to the hike described. The configuration defines the trail as a loop, an out-and-back (taking you in and out via the same route), a figure-eight, or a balloon. As the mileage is for the total hike, it is measured round-trip.

HIKING TIME

Unlike distance, which is a real, measured number, hiking time is an estimate. Every hiker has a different pace. Three miles per hour is a general rule of thumb from this hiker-author's point of view. That pace typically allows time for taking photos, for dawdling and admiring views, and for alternating stretches of hills and descents. When deciding whether or not to follow a particular trail in this guidebook, consider your own pace, weather, general physical condition, and energy level that day.

HIGHLIGHTS

The author provides a capsule list of the main attractions, such as a waterfall or a historical site, that draw hikers to this trail.

ELEVATION

In each trail's opener, you will see the elevation at the trailhead and another figure for the peak height on that route. For routes that entail significant inclines and declines, the full hike profile will also include a complete elevation profile (see above).

ACCESS

Fees or permits needed to hike the trail are indicated here, and I note if there are none. The hours the trail is open are also listed here.

MAPS

Here, I indicate where to obtain an additional map for this hike.

FACILITIES

For planning your hike, it's helpful to know what to expect at the trailhead or nearby in terms of restrooms, phones, water, and other niceties.

WHEELCHAIR ACCESS

For each hike, you will readily see whether or not it is feasible for the enjoyment of outdoor enthusiasts who use a wheelchair.

COMMENTS

Here you will find assorted nuggets of information, such as whether or not your dog is allowed on the trails.

CONTACTS

You'll find phone numbers and websites here to check trail conditions or to answer other questions.

Overview, Route Details, Nearby Attractions, & Directions

Each profile contains a complete narrative of the hike: "Overview" gives you a quick summary of what to expect on that trail. "Route Details" guides you on the hike, start to finish. "Nearby Attractions" suggests other area sites that you might like, such as restaurants, museums, or other trails. "Directions" will get you to the trailhead from a well-known road or highway.

Weather

Fall is the best season to hike in southeastern Michigan, not only because of the brilliant foliage but also because the temperatures are more moderate, the flies and mosquitoes are far less of a nuisance, and summer overgrowth has receded from the trails.

Early winter, before the heavy snow and frigid temperatures arrive, also can be enjoyable; evergreens stand more prominent in the woods, and topographical features become more noticeable without the foliage. And there are fewer hikers and bikers on the trails.

Early to mid-spring can be problematic. Many trails pass through and around wetlands, so it's not uncommon to find trails unwalkable or even closed because of flooding. Mid- to late spring is the best time to see wildflowers in full bloom.

For the most part, skip hiking in the summer. The flies and mosquitoes are especially bad and can make hiking a miserable experience.

DETROIT			
MONTH	HI TEMP	LO TEMP	RAIN
January	18°F	31°F	1.9"
February	20°F	34°F	1.9"
March	29°F	45°F	2.5"
April	38°F	58°F	3.0"
May	49°F	70°F	3.0"
June	59°F	79°F	3.6"
July	64°F	83°F	3.2"
August	62°F	81°F	3.1"
September	54°F	74°F	3.3"
October	43°F	61°F	2.2"

DETROIT			
MONTH	**HI TEMP**	**LO TEMP**	**RAIN**
November	34°F	48°F	2.7"
December	23°F	36°F	2.5"

ANN ARBOR			
MONTH	**HI TEMP**	**LO TEMP**	**RAIN**
January	17°F	30°F	2.2"
February	19°F	34°F	2.0"
March	27°F	45°F	2.8"
April	37°F	58°F	3.4"
May	48°F	70°F	3.0"
June	58°F	79°F	3.4"
July	62°F	83°F	3.2"
August	61°F	81°F	3.7"
September	53°F	74°F	3.4"
October	42°F	61°F	2.5"
November	32°F	47°F	3.0"
December	22°F	35°F	2.8"

Water

How much is enough? Well, one simple physiological fact should convince you to err on the side of excess when deciding how much water to pack—a hiker walking steadily in 90° heat needs approximately 10 quarts of fluid per day. That's 2.5 gallons. A good rule of thumb is to hydrate prior to your hike, carry (and drink) 6 ounces of water for every mile you plan to hike, and hydrate again after the hike. For most people, the pleasures of hiking make carrying water a relatively minor price to pay to remain safe and healthy. So pack more water than you anticipate needing even for short hikes.

If you are tempted to drink "found water," do so with extreme caution. Many ponds and lakes encountered by hikers are fairly stagnant and taste terrible, plus they present inherent risks for thirsty trekkers. Giardia parasites contaminate many water sources and cause the dreaded intestinal giardiasis that can last for weeks after ingestion. For information, visit The Centers for Disease Control website at **cdc.gov/parasites/giardia.**

In any case, effective treatment is essential before using any water source found along the trail. Boiling water for 2–3 minutes is always a safe measure for camping, but day hikers can consider iodine tablets, approved chemical mixes, filtration units rated for giardia, and UV filtration. Some of these methods (for example, filtration with an added carbon filter) remove bad tastes typical in stagnant water, while others add their own taste. Carry a means of purification to help in a pinch, if you realize you have underestimated your consumption needs.

Clothing

Weather, unexpected trail conditions, fatigue, injury, extended hiking duration, and wrong turns can individually or collectively turn a great outing into a very uncomfortable one at best—and a life-threatening one at worst. Thus, proper attire plays a key role in staying comfortable and, sometimes, staying alive. Here are some helpful guidelines.

★ Choose silk, wool, or synthetics for maximum comfort in all of your hiking attire—from hats to socks and in between. Cotton is fine if the weather remains dry and stable, but you won't be happy if it gets wet.

★ Always wear a hat, or at least tuck one into your day pack or hitch it to your belt. Hats offer all-weather sun and wind protection as well as warmth if it turns cold.

★ Be ready to layer up or down as the day progresses and the mercury rises or falls. Today's outdoor wear makes layering easy, with such designs as jackets that convert to vests and zip-off or button-up legs.

★ Wear hiking boots or sturdy hiking sandals with toe protection.

Flip-flopping on a paved path in an urban botanical garden is one thing, but never hike a trail in open sandals or casual sneakers. Your bones and arches need support, and your skin needs protection.

★ Pair that footwear with good socks! If you prefer not to sheath your feet when wearing hiking sandals, tuck the socks into your day pack; you may need them if the temperature plummets or if you hit rocky turf and pebbles begin to irritate your feet. And, in an emergency, if you have lost your gloves, you can adapt the socks into mittens.

★ Don't leave rainwear behind, even if the day dawns clear and sunny. Tuck into your day pack, or tie around your waist, a jacket that is breathable and either water-resistant or waterproof. Investigate different choices at your local outdoors retailer. If you are a frequent hiker, ideally you'll have more than one rainwear weight, material, and style in your closet to protect you in all seasons in your regional climate and hiking microclimates.

Essential Gear

Today you can buy outdoor vests that have up to 20 pockets shaped and sized to carry everything from toothpicks to binoculars, or if you don't aspire to feel like a burro, you can neatly stow all of these items in your day pack or backpack. The following list showcases never-hike-without-them items.

★ *Water* (As emphasized more than once in this book, bring more than you think you will drink; depending on your destination, you may want to bring a water bottle and iodine or filter for purifying water in the wilderness in case you run out.)

★ *Map and high-quality compass* (Even if you know the terrain from previous hikes, don't leave home without these tools.)

★ *Pocketknife* and/or multitool

★ *Flashlight* or headlamp with extra bulb and batteries

★ *Windproof matches* and/or a lighter, as well as a fire starter

★ *Extra food* (trail mix, granola bars, or other high-energy foods)

★ *Extra clothes* (raingear, warm hat, gloves, and change of socks and shirt)

★ *Whistle* (This little gadget will be your best friend in an emergency.)

★ *Insect repellent* (For some areas and seasons, this is vital.)

★ *Sunscreen* (Note the expiration date on the tube or bottle; it's usually embossed on the top.)

First-aid Kit

In addition to the items in the previous section, those following may appear overwhelming for a day hike. But any paramedic will tell you that the products listed here, in alphabetical order, are just the basics. The reality of hiking is that you can be out for a week of backpacking and acquire only a mosquito bite—or you can hike for an hour, slip, and suffer a bleeding abrasion or broken bone. Fortunately, these items will collapse into a very small space, and convenient, prepackaged kits are available at your pharmacy and on the Internet.

★ Ace bandages or Spenco joint wraps

★ Antibiotic ointment (Neosporin or the generic equivalent)

★ Athletic tape

★ Band-Aids

★ Benadryl or the generic equivalent diphenhydramine (in case of allergic reactions)

★ Blister kit (such as Moleskin/Spenco Second Skin)

★ Butterfly-closure bandages

★ Epinephrine in a prefilled syringe (for people known to have severe allergic reactions to such things as bee stings, usually available by prescription only)

★ Gauze (one roll and a half dozen 4-by-4-inch pads)

★ Hydrogen peroxide or iodine

★ Ibuprofen or acetaminophen

Consider your intended terrain and the number of hikers in your party before you exclude any article cited above. A botanical garden stroll may not inspire you to carry a complete kit, but anything beyond that warrants precaution.

When hiking alone, you should always be prepared for a medical need. And if you are a twosome or with a group, one or more people in your party should be equipped with first-aid material.

General Safety

The following tips may have the familiar ring of your mother's voice as you take note of them.

★ *Always let someone know* where you will be hiking and how long you expect to be gone. It's a good idea to give that person a copy of your route, particularly if you are headed into any isolated area. Let them know when you return.

★ *Always sign in and out of any trail registers provided.* Don't hesitate to comment on the trail condition if space is provided; that's your opportunity to alert others to any problems you encounter.

★ *Do not count on a cell phone for your safety.* Reception may be spotty or nonexistent on the trail, even on an urban walk embraced by towering trees.

★ *Always carry food and water,* even for a short hike. And bring more water than you think you will need. (I cannot say that often enough!)

★ *Stay on designated trails.* Even on the most clearly marked trails, there is usually a point where you have to stop and consider in which direction to head. If you become disoriented, don't panic. As soon as you think you may be off track, stop, assess your current direction, and then retrace your steps to the point where you went astray. Using a map, a compass, and this book, and keeping in mind what you have passed thus far, reorient yourself, and trust your judgment on which way to continue. If you become absolutely unsure of how to continue, return to your vehicle the way you came in. Should you become completely lost and have no idea how to return to the trailhead, remaining in place along the trail and waiting for help is most often the best option for adults and always the best option for children.

★ *Always carry a whistle.* It may be a lifesaver (or at least a major stress reducer) if you do become lost or sustain an injury.

★ *Be especially careful when crossing streams.* Whether you are fording the stream or crossing on a log, make every step count. If you have any doubt about maintaining your balance on a log, ford the stream instead; use a trekking pole or stout stick for balance and face upstream as you cross. If a stream seems too deep to ford, turn back. Whatever is on the other side is not worth risking your life.

★ *Be careful at overlooks.* While these areas may provide spectacular views, they are potentially hazardous. Stay back from the edge of outcrops and be absolutely sure of your footing; a misstep can mean a nasty and possibly fatal fall.

★ *Standing dead trees and storm-damaged living trees pose a real hazard to hikers.* These trees may have loose or broken limbs that could fall at any time. While walking beneath trees, and when choosing a spot to rest or enjoy your snack, look up!

★ *Know the symptoms of hypothermia.* Shivering and forgetfulness are the two most common indicators of this stealthy killer. Hypothermia can occur at any elevation, even in the summer, especially when the hiker is wearing lightweight cotton clothing. If symptoms present themselves, get to shelter, hot liquids, and dry clothes as soon as possible.

★ *Ask questions.* State forest and park employees are there to help. It's a lot easier to ask advice beforehand, and it will help you avoid a mishap away from civilization when it's too late to amend an error.

★ *Most important of all, take along your brain.* A cool, calculating mind is the single most important asset on the trail. Think before you act. Watch your step. Plan ahead. Avoiding accidents before they happen is the best way to ensure a rewarding and relaxing hike.

Watchwords for Flora & Fauna

Hikers should remain aware of the following concerns regarding plant- and wildlife, described in alphabetical order.

BLACK BEARS: Though attacks by black bears are virtually unheard of, the sight or approach of a bear can give anyone a start. It would be extremely rare to encounter a black bear while hiking in southeast Michigan, but if you do, remain calm and never run away. Make loud noises to scare off the bear and back away slowly. In primitive and remote areas, assume bears are present; in more developed sites, check on the current bear situation prior to hiking. Most encounters are food related, as bears have an exceptional sense of smell and not particularly discriminating tastes. While this is of greater concern to backpackers and campers, on a day hike, you may plan a lunchtime picnic or munch on a power bar or other snack from time to time. So remain aware and alert.

BLACK FLIES: Though certainly a pest and maddening annoyance, the worst a black fly will cause is an itchy welt. They are most active from late May into August during the day, and especially before thunderstorms, as well as during the morning and evening hours. Insect repellent has some effect, though the only way to keep them from swarming is to keep moving.

MOSQUITOES: Insect repellent and/or repellent-impregnated clothing are the only simple methods to ward off these pests. Repellents are a must when hiking in June, July, and even into mid-August. Mosquitoes are particularly bad along the trails that pass in and around wetlands and lakes. In some areas, mosquitoes are known to carry the West Nile virus, so all due caution should be taken to avoid their bites.

POISON IVY & SUMAC: Recognizing and avoiding poison ivy and sumac are the most effective ways to prevent the painful, itchy rashes associated with these plants. Poison ivy occurs as a vine or groundcover, three leaflets to a leaf, and is likely to be found among most of the trails in this book. Poison sumac flourishes in swampland but also can be found near swamps, shrubby wet depressions, and meadows. Each leaf has 7–13 leaflets.

Urushiol, the oil in the sap of these plants, is responsible for the rash. Within 14 hours of exposure, raised lines and/or blisters will appear on the affected area, accompanied by a terrible itch. Refrain from scratching because bacteria under your fingernails can cause an infection. Wash and dry the affected area thoroughly, applying a calamine lotion to help dry out the rash. If itching or blistering is severe, seek medical attention. If you do come into contact with one of these plants, remember that oil-contaminated clothes, pets, or hiking gear can easily cause an irritating rash on you or someone else, so wash not only any exposed parts of your body but also clothes, gear, and pets if applicable.

SNAKES: Rattlesnakes, cottonmouths, copperheads, and corals are among the most common venomous snakes in the United States, and hibernation season is typically October–April. In the region described in this book, you will possibly encounter the massasauga (*Sistrurus catenatus)* rattlesnake, the only poisonous snake native to the region. In areas where they are common, parks have posted warning signs. However, the snakes you most likely will see while hiking will be nonvenomous species and subspecies. The best rule is to leave all snakes alone, give them a wide berth as you hike past, and make sure any hiking companions (including dogs) do the same.

When hiking, stick to well-used trails and wear over-the-ankle boots and loose-fitting long pants. Rattlesnakes like to bask in the sun and won't bite unless threatened. Do not step or put your hands where you cannot see, and avoid wandering around in the dark. Step onto logs and rocks, never over them, and be especially careful when climbing rocks. Always avoid walking through dense brush or willow thickets.

TICKS: Ticks are often found on brush and tall grass, where they seem to be waiting to hitch a ride on a warm-blooded passerby. Adult ticks are most active April into May and again October into November. Among the varieties of ticks, the black-legged tick, commonly called the deer tick, is the primary carrier of Lyme disease. Wear light-colored clothing, so ticks can be spotted before they make it to the skin. And be sure to visually check your hair, back of neck, armpits, and socks at the end of the hike. During your post-hike shower, take a moment to do a more complete body check. For ticks that are already embedded, removal with tweezers is best. Use disinfectant solution on the wound.

Hunting

Separate rules, regulations, and licenses govern the various hunting types and related seasons. Many trails in the state recreation areas pass through areas open to hunting. Signs along the trail designate the areas. Hikers are not prohibited from walking the trails during hunting season. However, hikers may wish to forgo their trips during the big-game seasons, when the woods suddenly seem filled with orange and camouflage. Many areas are open to hunting from mid-September through the end of March. Hikers are most likely to encounter hunters during firearms season for deer, from mid- to late November.

For safety reasons, I would suggest avoiding hiking during this time; if you must hike, wear bright orange to stand out to hunters. Muzzle-loading season follows from early to mid-December, and small game hunting extends until the end of March.

Regulations

⭑ Carry out what you carry in. Practice "leave no trace" camping and hiking.

⭑ Observe and enjoy wildlife and plants, but leave them undisturbed.

⭑ Removing trees, shrubs, wildflowers, grasses, or other vegetation is illegal. Except in wildlife food plots, this does not include picking mushrooms, berries, and edible fruits and nuts for personal use.

Trail Etiquette

Always treat the trail, wildlife, and fellow hikers with respect. Here are some reminders.

⭑ *Plan ahead in order to be self-sufficient at all times;* carry necessary supplies for changes in weather or other conditions. A well-executed trip is a satisfaction to you and to others.

⭑ *Hike on open trails only.*

⭑ *Respect trail and road closures* (ask if not sure), avoid possible trespassing on private land, and obtain all permits and authorization as required. Also, leave gates as you found them or as marked.

⭑ *Be courteous to other hikers,* bikers, equestrians, and others you encounter on the trails.

⭑ *Never spook animals.* An unannounced approach, a sudden movement, or a loud noise startles most animals. A surprised animal can be dangerous to you, to others, and to itself. Give them plenty of space.

★ *Observe the* YIELD *signs* that are displayed around the region's trailheads and backcountry. They advise hikers to yield to horses, and bikers yield to both horses and hikers. A common courtesy on hills is that hikers and bikers yield to any uphill traffic. When encountering mounted riders or horse packers, hikers can courteously step off the trail, on the downhill side if possible. Speak to the riders before they reach you and do not dart behind trees. You are less spooky if the horse can see and hear you. Resist the urge to pet horses unless you are invited to do so.

★ *Leave only footprints.* Be sensitive to the ground beneath you. This also means staying on the existing trail and not blazing any new trails.

★ *Be sure to pack out what you pack in.* No one likes to see the trash someone else has left behind.

Tips on Hiking in Greater Detroit and Ann Arbor

Before heading out to hike, check with the park office about possible trail closings and conditions. In the spring, in particular, trails can be closed because of flooding or lack of seasonal maintenance. Unfortunately, these closings are generally not posted at the trailhead or noted on park websites. I've encountered closed trails on several outings. Trails can also be quite muddy in the spring; dress appropriately.

Picking up a map or printing one from the park website cannot be stressed enough. I've frequently encountered uprooted or missing trail markers at confusing intersections. Trail maintenance is spotty at state park and recreation areas.

If you're seeking solitude, it's best to hike on weekdays. Many trails in state recreation areas are popular with mountain bikers, especially on the weekends. A constant parade of bikers can mar your hiking experience. Your best bet is to hike these trails on weekdays. Bikers, for the most part, are courteous and will warn you if they're coming up behind you. Scouting and other groups frequently use trails on the weekends for special events and outings.

Getting to most of these hiking destinations requires traveling some very busy roads in metropolitan Detroit and Ann Arbor. To avoid traffic congestion during morning and afternoon rush hours, plan your hikes in late mornings and early afternoons.

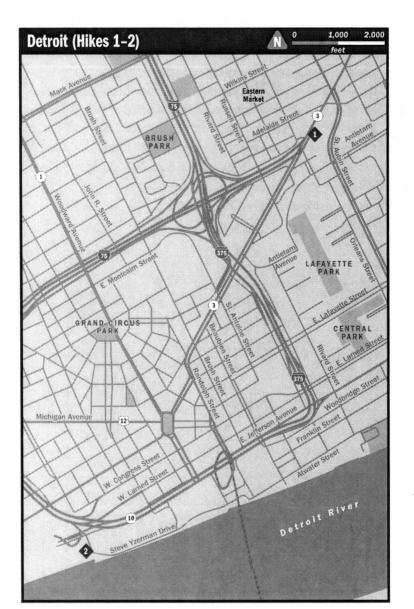

Detroit (Hikes 1–2)

N
0   1,000   2,000
feet

Mack Avenue

Wilkins Street

Eastern Market

Brush Street

75

BRUSH PARK

Russell Street

Rivard Street

Adelaide Street

3

1

Antietam Avenue

St. Aubin Street

1

John R. Street

Woodward Avenue

Orleans Street

76

E. Montcalm Street

375

Antietam Avenue

LAFAYETTE PARK

3

St. Antoine Street

Beaubien Street

E. Lafayette Street

CENTRAL PARK

Rivard Street

E. Larned Street

GRAND CIRCUS PARK

Brush Street

Randolph Street

375

Michigan Avenue

12

Woodbridge Street

E. Jefferson Avenue

Franklin Street

W. Congress Street

W. Larned Street

Atwater Street

10

Steve Yzerman Drive

2

Detroit River

Detroit

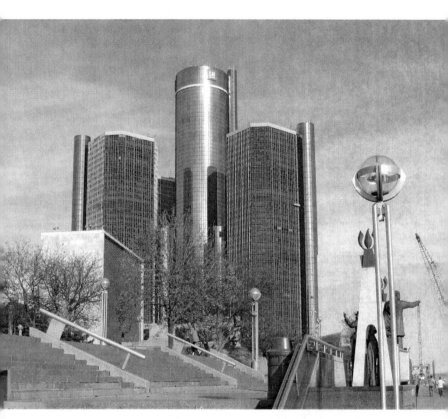

A VIEW OF THE RENAISSANCE CENTER FROM THE DETROIT RIVERWALK

Dequindre Cut Greenway

SCENERY: ★ ★ ★
TRAIL CONDITION: ★ ★ ★ ★ ★
CHILDREN: ★ ★ ★ ★ ★
DIFFICULTY: ★
SOLITUDE: ★ ★

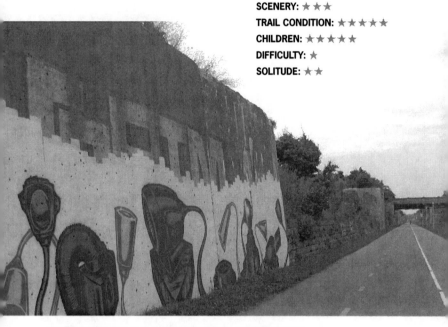

GRAFFITI-LIKE ART ALONG THE DEQUINDRE CUT GREENWAY

GPS TRAILHEAD COORDINATES: N42° 20.827' W83° 2.134'

DISTANCE & CONFIGURATION: 2.6-mile out-and-back

HIKING TIME: About 1 hour or less

HIGHLIGHTS: Graffiti art, Lafayette Towers, Eastern Market

ELEVATION: 612 feet at trailhead, with no significant rise

ACCESS: Daily, 6 a.m.–10 p.m.; no fees or permits required

MAPS: At **detroitriverfront.org/dequindre**

FACILITIES: Restrooms, picnic areas at William G. Milliken State Park and Harbor

WHEELCHAIR ACCESS: Yes

COMMENTS: While the trail is well lit and there are emergency phones, it's best to avoid the trail after dark. Most of the trail runs below street level, making it isolated from activity in the surrounding neighborhoods.

CONTACTS: 313-566-8200; **detroitriverfront.org**

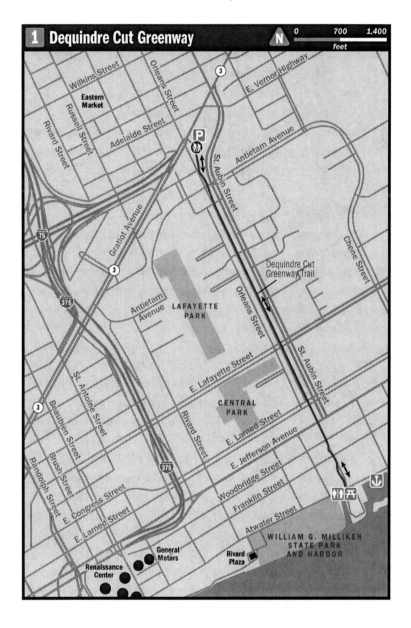

1 Dequindre Cut Greenway

N

0   700   1,400

feet

Wilkins Street

Orleans Street

E. Vernor Highway

Eastern Market

Russell Street

Rivard Street

Adelaide Street

Antietam Avenue

St. Aubin Street

Gratiot Avenue

Chene Street

Dequindre Cut Greenway Trail

Orleans Street

Antietam Avenue

LAFAYETTE PARK

St. Antoine Street

E. Lafayette Street

St. Aubin Street

Beaubien Street

CENTRAL PARK

Rivard Street

E. Larned Street

Brush Street

E. Jefferson Avenue

Randolph Street

E. Congress Street

E. Larned Street

Woodbridge Street

Franklin Street

Atwater Street

WILLIAM G. MILLIKEN STATE PARK AND HARBOR

General Motors

Rivard Plaza

Renaissance Center

Overview

The Dequindre Cut Greenway connects the Detroit RiverWalk at William G. Milliken State Park and Harbor, the only urban site in Michigan's state park system, to the city's historic Eastern Market. The Dequindre Cut makes for an ideal leisurely walk before or after a trip to the market or a visit to the riverfront. The market comes alive on Saturday mornings, when farmers from around the state set up stands to sell fresh produce, herbs, flowers, and meat.

Route Details

Not too long ago, commuter trains ran along the 60-foot-wide swath that cuts below street level from Eastern Market to Rivertown, a popular nightclub and restaurant area just east of the downtown business district. The commuter trains are long gone and Rivertown is no longer a thriving entertainment center, but the Dequindre Cut is finding new life as an urban greenway.

Opened in 2009, the Dequindre Cut derives its name from the stretch of the old Grand Trunk Railroad line that dropped 25 feet as it approached downtown Detroit near Eastern Market. The trail follows the same path, running primarily below street level. It's been redeveloped, of course, with a 20-foot-wide pavement replacing the railroad. Still, you get a sense of the path of the old rail line.

Perhaps the most convenient access is off Gratiot Avenue at Eastern Market. A dirt parking lot is located on the south side of Gratiot Avenue/M-3, east of St. Aubin Street. No signs point to the parking lot, but as you pull into the lot (a vacant lot, really), you'll see a large sign marking the Dequindre Cut Greenway. The entrance is to the left of the sign; a paved ramp descends to the trail.

You can also access the trail from Lafayette Boulevard and from Woodbridge and Atwater streets at the trail's southern entrance. No parking is at the Lafayette entrance. Parking is available along both Woodbridge and Atwater streets. You can also park in the public lot at Rivard Plaza on Atwater Street and then walk a few blocks east to the trail entrance.

Whether you begin the trail at points south or north, it's a straight shot in either direction. The Gratiot Avenue entrance is an ideal starting point because you can enjoy Eastern Market, especially on Saturdays, its main day of business. Tens of thousands of shoppers descend on the market to buy everything from vegetables and fruits to flowers and herbs to pies and cakes, and a whole lot more. Shops and restaurants surround the open-air sheds and sell wine, spices, and antiques. Most of them are open weekdays as well.

From the Gratiot Avenue entrance, you'll head due south. Signposts mark distances. Walking below street level, in a parklike setting, makes for an unusual experience. As you head south, you'll be able see the steeples of churches above the cement walls on either side. Continuing south, you'll notice on your right the towers of Lafayette Park, a residential and park complex planned by Mies van der Rohe. Lafayette Park was created as part of an urban renewal project in the 1950s.

The paved path is 20 feet wide with lanes marked for walkers and bicyclists. The rest of the swath is natural grasses and has been reserved for possible rail transit in the future. The stretch has been spruced up with newly planted trees and flowers. Park benches, streetlights, and emergency phones line the route as well.

One of the outstanding features of this urban trail is the graffiti along the cement walls and the pillars of overpasses. During the years after the railroad abandoned the line, the corridor became a haven for the homeless and a canvas for guerilla painters, who remade the corridor into an unofficial art park. The graffiti is ever changing and, to locals, remains part of the charm of this urban trail. Redevelopment of the rail line into a greenway has chased away the homeless. The trail is well lit, and emergency phones are posted along the route. Detroit police officers patrol the cut regularly. In the warmer months, the trail is busy with bicyclists, runners, and families.

After crossing the last of the overpasses (Jefferson Avenue), the trail opens up to the streetscape. An extension opened in 2010 with plazas between Woodbridge and Franklin streets, and Franklin and Atwater streets. They're nicely landscaped with flowers, trees, and benches. On the opposite side of Atwater Street are William G. Milliken State Park and Harbor and the Detroit River. The park includes picnic tables, grassy knolls, benches, and restrooms. It's a great vantage point to watch freighters and recreational boats pass by.

To return to the Gratiot Avenue entrance, simply turn around and head north, retracing your steps.

Nearby Attractions

At the southern end of the Dequindre Cut Greenway, William G. Milliken State Park and Harbor offers an up-close view of the Detroit River and connects to the city's popular RiverWalk. Formerly Tricentennial State Park, Milliken occupies just 31 acres, but it offers a picnic area, restroom facilities, and a 52-slip marina.

Directions

From Detroit, take I-75 south to Mack Avenue, Exit 52. Continue straight on Chrysler Drive and turn left on Wilkins Street. Cross over I-375 and turn right onto Chrysler Drive (the service drive goes both directions below Wilkins); follow about 0.4 miles to Russell Street. Turn right on Russell Street. Turn left on Gratiot Avenue and follow about 0.5 miles. Parking for the Dequindre Cut Greenway is on your right, just past St. Joseph Catholic Church (also on your right).

From Ann Arbor, take I-94 east about 33 miles to US 10 (the Lodge), Exit 215A. Follow US 10 south toward downtown Detroit. Merge onto I-75 north, Exit 2A, toward Flint. Exit left onto M-3/Gratiot Avenue, Exit 51. Merge left onto Gratiot Avenue. Parking for the Dequindre Cut Greenway is about 0.5 miles on your right, beyond St. Joseph Catholic Church.

Detroit RiverWalk

SCENERY: ★ ★ ★ ★ ★
TRAIL CONDITION: ★ ★ ★ ★ ★
CHILDREN: ★ ★ ★ ★ ★
DIFFICULTY: ★
SOLITUDE: ★

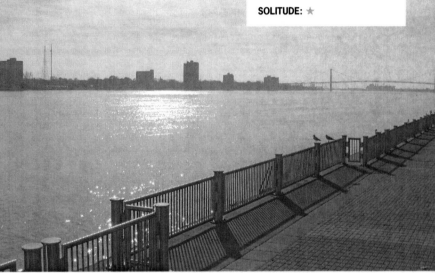

LOOKING ACROSS THE DETROIT RIVER TO WINDSOR, ONTARIO

GPS TRAILHEAD COORDINATES: N42° 19.541' W83° 3.166'

DISTANCE & CONFIGURATION: 2-mile out-and-back

HIKING TIME: About 1 hour or less

HIGHLIGHTS: Detroit River; skyline views of Windsor, Ontario, Canada; Hart Plaza; General Motors global headquarters

ELEVATION: 583 feet at trailhead, with no significant rise

ACCESS: Daily, 6 a.m.–10 p.m.; no fees or permits required

MAPS: At **detroitriverfront.org**

FACILITIES: Restrooms (seasonal), picnic areas, bike rentals, café

WHEELCHAIR ACCESS: Yes

COMMENTS: The path can be very crowded during lunchtime and summer evenings. Watch out for bicyclists.

CONTACTS: 313-566-8200; **detroitriverfront.org**

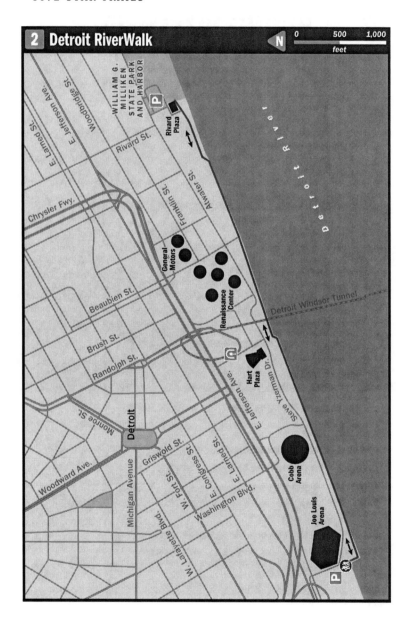

Overview

One of the newest developments in downtown, the Detroit RiverWalk opens up a vast stretch of the riverfront to the public. The well-maintained path offers panoramic views of the scenic Detroit River and the Windsor skyline, and it passes directly by the General Motors global headquarters at the Renaissance Center.

Route Details

Strolling along the Detroit RiverWalk, you may find it hard to believe that the city didn't realize until very recently what a jewel the turquoise-shaded river is. Once home to industrial plants, silos, and other buildings, much of the riverfront is being converted into promenades, parks, and public spaces.

The crown jewel, of course, is the Detroit RiverWalk, an expansive walkway that runs along the river and will eventually stretch 5.5 miles from the Ambassador Bridge on the city's western edge to Belle Isle, an island park on the east.

More than half of the walk has been completed, though portions remain separated by vacant remnants of the past. The best bet is to start the Detroit RiverWalk at its western edge near Joe Louis Arena, and you can park along the street running next to the stadium. The promenade parallels the Detroit River with separate lanes for walkers, hikers, bicyclists, and inline skaters. Expect to find plenty of people crowding the promenade during the warmer months, as well as fishermen lined along the rails, casting their nets into the fast-moving river.

Heading east along the riverfront, the promenade passes below Philip A. Hart Plaza, an open, mostly hard-surfaced park. This is the approximate landing site of Antoine de la Mothe Cadillac, who in 1701 founded the settlement that eventually became Detroit. Today the park is the site of festivals throughout the summer and is noteworthy for several sculptures, including a statue of Cadillac, as well as the Horace E. Dodge and Son Memorial Fountain, designed by Isamu Noguchi.

The Renaissance Center, the global home of General Motors, will catch your attention as you continue east. You'll find plenty of people sitting along the concrete steps leading up to the Winter Garden, and in the summer months, diners enjoy their meals at the outdoor patio at Andiamo, a well-known Detroit restaurant. The tallest and central tower is home to the Detroit Marriott at the Renaissance Center, the tallest all-hotel skyscraper in the Western Hemisphere. The surrounding four towers are occupied by GM and other automotive-related companies.

The promenade continues to Rivard Plaza, home to a Great Lakes–themed carousel, a water-jet fountain and pool, a map of the Detroit River system (made of granite), and a vertical glass map of the entire St. Lawrence Seaway. Walkers also will find a bike rental store, a concession stand selling Michigan-inspired fare, and restroom facilities. There are plenty of tables and chairs for outdoor dining.

At the plaza's eastern edge is William G. Milliken State Park and Harbor, formerly known as Tricentennial State Park, Michigan's only state park in an urban area. The 31-acre park contains a marina, and a 63-foot conical lighthouse marks the entrance. Retrace your steps along the river back to the starting point.

If you're more adventurous and wish to extend your walk beyond the state park, continue walking along Atwater Street. Although this stretch veers from the riverfront, it is part of the RiverWalk. You'll pass the southern entrance of the Dequindre Cut Greenway as you head due east. The RiverWalk, however, officially ends—for now—at Chene Street, beyond the entrance of Chene Park. To reach the next completed stretch of the RiverWalk, continue walking another block or so along Atwater Street to Joseph Campau Street. Turn right and head past the gatehouse to the riverfront. The promenade continues past Stroh River Place, the former Omni hotel, and the United Auto Workers–General Motors offices to Mount Elliott Park. Adding this stretch creates about a 3.5-mile one-way trek from the beginning point at Joe Louis Arena.

Nearby Attractions

GM's Winter Garden offers restaurants, shops, and other services. Coach Insignia, the restaurant atop the RenCen, is open in the evenings for dinner. The restaurant offers a panoramic view of the city, the river, and neighboring Windsor, Ontario. The glass elevator to the 72nd floor runs up the outside of the structure. It's about a 0.5-mile walk from Hart Plaza to the city's new center, Campus Martius, which features a small park with an outdoor café. In the summer, there are concerts, and in the winter, the grassy area is turned into an ice-skating rink.

Directions

From downtown, the RiverWalk is accessible from Hart Plaza right off Jefferson Avenue on the riverfront. To walk from one end to the other, start at either Rivard Plaza on the eastern end or at Joe Louis Arena on the west end. Heading east on Jefferson from Woodward Avenue, past the Renaissance Center, turn right onto Rivard Street. Turn left onto Atwater Street. A parking lot will be on your right. To reach the entrance near Joe Louis, head west on Jefferson Avenue and drive past the Renaissance Center, Hart Plaza, Cobo Center, and Joe Louis Arena. Third Street is immediately after Joe Louis. Turn left on Third Street. Parking is available along Third Street and Steve Yzerman Drive, a service drive to Joe Louis that runs parallel to the river.

From Ann Arbor, take US 23 north/M-14 east to Plymouth. M-14 becomes I-96. Continue about 20 miles on eastbound I-96 toward Detroit. Follow signs for M-10/Civic-Cobo Center. Merge onto M-10 and continue toward Civic Center/Cobo Center. Take Exit 1A, West Jefferson Avenue. Go straight, crossing Jefferson onto Third Street. Parking is available along Third Street and Steve Yzerman Drive, the service drive to Joe Louis and Cobo Center.

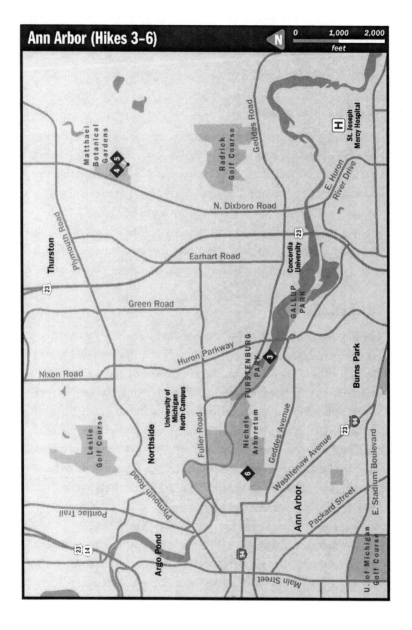

Ann Arbor (Hikes 3–6)

N

0   1,000   2,000

feet

Matthaei Botanical Gardens

Radrick Golf Course

Geddes Road

H

St. Joseph Mercy Hospital

4 5

N. Dixboro Road

E. Huron River Drive

Thurston

Plymouth Road

23

Earhart Road

23

Concordia University

Green Road

GALLUP PARK

Huron Parkway

FURSTENBURG PARK

3

Burns Park

Nixon Road

University of Michigan North Campus

Northside

Fuller Road

Nichols Arboretum

Geddes Avenue

Washtenaw Avenue

23

14

Leslie Golf Course

6

23

14

Pontiac Trail

Plymouth Road

Argo Pond

14

Packard Street

Ann Arbor

E. Stadium Boulevard

Main Street

14

U. of Michigan Golf Course

Ann Arbor

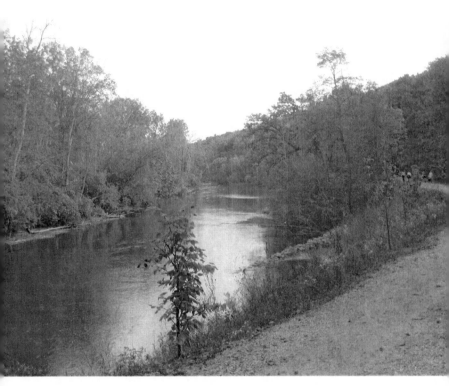

THE HURON RIVER SNAKES ALONG A TRAIL AT NICHOLS ABORETUM.

3 # Gallup Park Loop and Spur

SCENERY: ★ ★
TRAIL CONDITION: ★ ★ ★ ★ ★
CHILDREN: ★ ★ ★ ★ ★
DIFFICULTY: ★
SOLITUDE: ★ ★

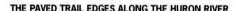

THE PAVED TRAIL EDGES ALONG THE HURON RIVER.

GPS TRAILHEAD COORDINATES: N42° 16.637' W83° 42.058'

DISTANCE & CONFIGURATION: 3.8-mile loop with a spur

HIKING TIME: About 1.5 hours

HIGHLIGHTS: Huron River, Geddes Pond, tiny river islands

ELEVATION: 750 feet at trailhead, with no significant rise

ACCESS: Daily, 7 a.m.–10 p.m.; no fees or permits required

MAPS: At the Ann Arbor Parks and Recreation, 100 N. Fifth Ave., 6th floor of City Hall, or **a2gov.org**

FACILITIES: Restrooms, picnic areas, playground, concession stand, kayak rentals

WHEELCHAIR ACCESS: Yes

COMMENTS: The path can be very crowded during lunchtime and on summer evenings. Watch out for bicyclists.

CONTACTS: 734-794-6230; **a2gov.org**

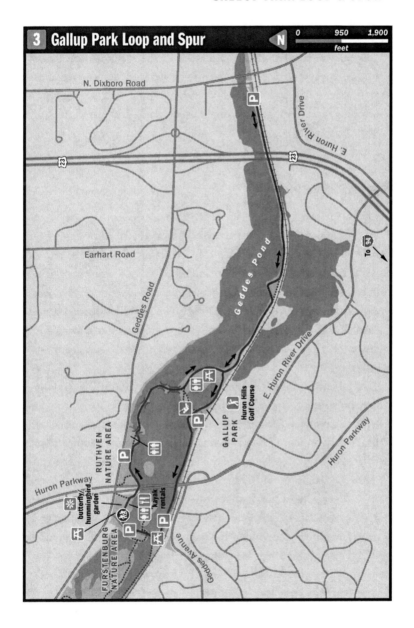

3 Gallup Park Loop and Spur

N

0   950   1,900
feet

N. Dixboro Road

E. Huron River Drive

23

23

Earhart Road

To

Geddes Road

Geddes Pond

E. Huron River Drive

RUTHVEN NATURE AREA

GALLUP PARK

Huron Hills Golf Course

Huron Parkway

Huron Parkway

butterfly/ hummingbird garden

kayak rentals

FURSTENBURG NATURE AREA

Geddes Avenue

Overview

This 69-acre park straddles both sides of the scenic Huron River, connecting from one side to the other over a series of tiny islands and bridges. The park is a well-known locale for walking, running, bicycling, and skating, with ample playgrounds and picnic areas to boot. Despite its popularity, the park remains an enjoyable place for a nice stroll.

Route Details

Gallup Park was dedicated in 1958 in memory of Eli A. Gallup, a superintendent of Ann Arbor parks. Although well known as a city park, it has also been part of the National Trail System since 1982.

Two trails—an inner loop and an outer loop—run parallel to one another as they circle this picturesque park north of downtown Ann Arbor near the Huron Hills Golf Course and the Ruthven Nature Area. The gentle, easy-to-follow trails loop around Geddes Pond and cross the Huron River, offering stretches of lovely scenery in an urban setting.

The inner loop is 1.4 miles long, and the slightly longer outer loop measures 1.7 miles. Either of these leisurely strolls can be extended with the Dixboro Mile, located at the park's far eastern end, or the Arboretum Mile at the western end. The inner and outer loops diverge as they cross the last of the bridges over the Huron River and reach the Gallup Youth Fishing Pond.

The trailhead stands about 100 feet from the parking lot. You'll see a large wooden sign marking the beginning of the trail system and providing information about the park. Picnic tables, grills, drinking fountains, and benches are scattered throughout the park, mostly near the river. The Dixboro Mile and a narrow stretch on the river's south side have no picnic facilities.

For the purposes of this hike, follow the outer loop, which adds a little more distance to the trek and includes the Dixboro Mile. Heading eastward, the paved path immediately passes a playground on one side and a canoe livery, concession stand, and restrooms on the other. The livery is one of two in Ann Arbor parks and offers kayak, canoe, rowboat, and pedal boat rentals, as well as organized river trips.

The path soon crosses under the Huron Parkway and runs parallel to Geddes Road. Around 0.2 miles, you'll pass a butterfly and hummingbird garden on the left. The first in a series of small wooden bridges begins at about the 0.3-mile mark. The path turns from pavement to wooden chips as it crosses three tiny narrow islands and connects to the park's south side.

The bridges reach the opposite shore at the Gallup Youth Fishing Pond and another picnic and playground area. Here, swing left, heading south and southeast to follow the outer loop to the intersection with the Dixboro Mile. You'll reach that intersection around the 1.1-mile mark. Bear left, following the trail due east to Dixboro Road, along the southern shoreline of the Huron River.

Along this stretch, the trail darts between the south shore of the Huron River and railroad tracks on the opposite side. Much of the shoreline is thinly lined with trees. Homes and at least one church are visible amid the wooded hills on the opposite banks. About 0.5 miles later, the path crosses underneath the two bridges—north- and southbound lanes of US 23.

The Dixboro Mile ends about 0.2 miles later near a small dam and a parking lot off Dixboro Road. The parking lot separates the trail from the road. A small overlook allows a closer glimpse of the river and dam. From this juncture, retrace your steps back in the opposite direction, heading due west.

You'll return to the outer loop and the Gallup Youth Fishing Pond around the 3-mile mark. From this juncture, the path passes a playground and a parking area. From here, it's about 0.5 miles to a long wooden bridge that leads back to the main parking lot. The path continues due westward largely along the riverfront, with a thin line of trees on one side and railroad tracks on the other. Scattered houses and the Huron Hills Golf Course are visible to the south. The path again crosses under the Huron Parkway overpass before reaching the bridge back to the main parking area.

Nearby Attractions

Just west of Gallup Park, the adjoining Furstenberg Nature Area offers 37 acres of wetlands, woodlands, prairie, and oak savannah. Paved and granular trails crisscross the prairie and woods, and a 0.3-mile-long boardwalk snakes through wetlands. An interpretive brochure explains numbered posts along the trails. A pedestrian bridge connects Gallup Park to the nature area.

Directions

From Detroit, follow I-94 west about 35 miles to Exit 180B, US 23 north. Follow US 23 about 4 miles to Exit 39, Geddes Road. Turn left on Geddes Road and follow it for about 1.3 miles. Geddes becomes Fuller Road after crossing Huron Parkway. The entrance to Gallup Park is on the left.

From Ann Arbor, at Huron and Main streets, head east on East Huron (I-94 Bus/US 23) about 0.7 miles to Glen Avenue. Turn left. At about 0.4 miles, Glen Avenue turns into Fuller Road. Follow it for about 2 miles to the park entrance, on your right, just before Huron Parkway.

4

Matthaei Botanical Gardens: Fleming Creek and Dix Pond Trails

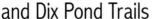

SCENERY: ★ ★ ★
TRAIL CONDITION: ★ ★ ★ ★
CHILDREN: ★ ★ ★
DIFFICULTY: ★ ★
SOLITUDE: ★ ★

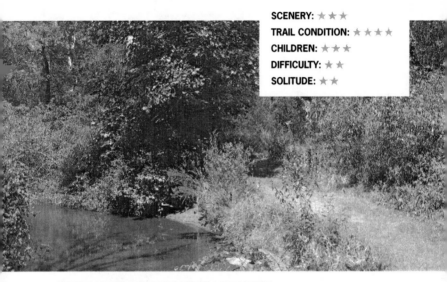

FLEMING CREEK SEPARATES VARIED LANDSCAPES.

GPS TRAILHEAD COORDINATES: N42° 17.991' W83° 39.651'

DISTANCE & CONFIGURATION: 1.6-mile loop

HIKING TIME: About 1 hour or less

HIGHLIGHTS: Woodlands, fields, Fleming Creek, ponds

ELEVATION: 790 feet at trailhead, with no significant rise

ACCESS: Daily, sunrise–sunset; no fees or permits required for grounds. Conservatory, garden shop, and visitor center Monday, Tuesday, and Thursday–Sunday, 10 a.m.–4:30 p.m.; Wednesday, 10 a.m.–8 p.m. Adults, $5; children 5–18, $2; free, children under 5

MAPS: In the visitor center and at **mbgna.umich.edu**

FACILITIES: Visitor center, conservatory, garden shop, restrooms

WHEELCHAIR ACCESS: Yes, in the conservatory and display gardens, as well as on the Sue Reichert Discovery Trail and on the Sam Graham Trees Trail, but not on the Dix Pond Trail.

COMMENTS: Dogs are not permitted except for guide dogs. Bicycles are not allowed on the trails. Do not handle snakes: the massasauga rattlesnake is frequently spotted on the grounds.

CONTACTS: 734-647-7600; **mbgna.umich.edu**

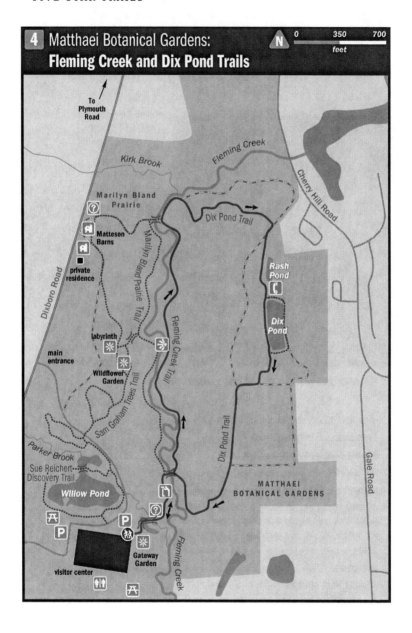

4 Matthaei Botanical Gardens: Fleming Creek and Dix Pond Trails

N   0   350   700
feet

To Plymouth Road

Fleming Creek

Kirk Brook

Cherry Hill Road

Marilyn Bland Prairie

Matteson Barns

private residence

Dixboro Road

Marilyn Bland Prairie Trail

Dix Pond Trail

Rash Pond

Dix Pond

labyrinth

main entrance

Fleming Creek Trail

Wildflower Garden

Sam Graham Trees Trail

Dix Pond Trail

Parker Brook

Sue Reichert Discovery Trail

Willow Pond

MATTHAEI BOTANICAL GARDENS

Gateway Garden

visitor center

Fleming Creek

Gale Road

Overview

The combination of five trails plus several remarkable gardens make Matthaei Botanical Gardens a worthy destination. Combining the Fleming Creek and Dix Pond trails creates a loop through a diverse landscape on the eastern section of the garden property, through old pastures being reclaimed by nature, into maturing forests, and past a pair of ponds that were once part of a gravel mining operation. Afterward, a stroll through the several gardens and the conservatory make for an enjoyable afternoon in spring, summer, or fall.

Route Details

Both the Fleming Creek and Dix Pond trails begin on the opposite side of the creek. To connect to them, hikers must follow a 0.1-mile stretch of the Sam Graham Trees Trail. The Fleming Creek Trail then follows the eastern bank of Fleming Creek for about 0.5 miles to a wooden bridge and then becomes the Dix Pond Trail. To begin this loop, find the trailhead just outside the visitor center and the Gateway Garden. The trailhead is easy to spot just beyond the garden gates at the constructed wetlands.

At the trailhead, follow the wide stone path along a row of white cedars around the constructed wetlands and across a 100-plus-foot-long wooden bridge to a dirt gravel path. (Note the sign on the bridge, on your right, warning of TINY FROG CROSSING.) At the end of the bridge, a trail kiosk (with an earthen roof) stands directly in front of you. Beyond the kiosk, the wide dirt trail passes a variety of trees, including notable silver maples and tulip trees marked by small signs. About the 0.2-mile mark, an observation deck overlooks Fleming Creek. You will see a musclewood tree on your left.

After crossing a small wooden bridge to the opposite side of the creek, turn left (north). The Fleming Creek Trail follows the meandering Fleming Creek, its banks lined with tall shade trees—cottonwoods, walnuts, burr oaks, and tamaracks. There are occasional breaks in the woods with short paths leading to openings along the creek.

Northward, the trail rises slightly to become a grassy path high above the water. Beyond the 0.5-mile mark, near a wooden bridge (the Marilyn Bland Prairie Trail begins on the opposite side of the creek), bear right along the flat trail. This is now the Dix Pond Trail. Occasionally, you can hear water gushing over rocks and slight drops in the creek.

Around the 0.7-mile mark, swing right, remaining on the same side of the creek, to continue along the Dix Pond Trail. From this juncture, the Dix Pond Trail stretches eastward, crossing woodlands and old pastures.

Burr oaks and hickory shagbark dominated the original landscape before farming and logging occurred. Some of those species, along with a variety of maples, remain. The trail eventually winds southward toward the gardens.

Quaking aspens dot the area around Rash and Dix ponds, which were part of a gravel mining operation more than 50 years ago, and cottonwoods flank the ponds. Scattered Scotch pines, Norway spruce, and eastern red cedars contrast the hardwoods found along much of the trail.

At about the 0.9-mile mark, the trail passes under a low-lying canopy of trees, creating a tunnellike effect. Tall pines line the trail here. About 0.2 miles later, you'll encounter an open stretch of field. Occasional fox sightings have been reported along the trail, and spotting a massasauga rattlesnake is not uncommon.

At about 1.5 miles, the trail crosses back over Fleming Creek at the juncture where the Sam Graham Trees Trail runs north and south. Retrace your footsteps back to the starting point at the constructed wetlands and Gateway Garden.

Before or after hiking the trails, steal some time in the gardens. They are home to a diverse—and sometimes changing—selection of perennials, herbs, ornamental plants, wildflowers, and trees, among other plants. Summer and early fall are peak bloom times for perennials and tropical annuals. The Gaffield Children's Garden features play spaces, trails, plants to touch, a digging pit, and a maze.

In its 10,000 square feet, the Conservatory contains more than 1,200 species from around the world. The Desert House includes barrel cacti, aloe, and agave species.

The gardens are named after a former University of Michigan regent, Frederick C. Matthaei Sr., and his wife, Mildred, who donated 200 acres to the university. The gardens encompass 300 acres overall, and much of the land was once used for farming and logging. Although farming ended decades ago, some old pastures are still recognizable, and nature is slowly reclaiming fields once grazed by sheep.

Nearby Attractions

While you're here, try the Marilyn Bland Prairie Trail as well (see page 44). Ann Arbor, about a 10-minute drive from the garden, is a very walkable city. Its compact downtown layout boasts top-notch restaurants, brewpubs, coffee shops, stores, and boutiques. There's plenty of entertainment, including the State and Michigan theaters, as well as the cultural attractions on the University of Michigan central campus. Ann Arbor is well known as the home of Zingerman's Deli, which serves thousands of made-to-order sandwiches with premium deli meats. The store also stocks an exceptional selection of farmhouse cheeses, estate-bottled olive oils, varietal vinegars, smoked fish, salami, coffee, and tea. Expect long lines at lunchtime.

Directions

From Detroit, exit I-94 at Exit 180B, US 23 north (Flint). Then exit US 23 at Geddes Road. Turn right onto Geddes Road. Continue east on Geddes Road for approximately 0.1 mile; then turn left onto Dixboro Road. The gardens will be on your right after approximately 2 miles.

From Ann Arbor, take US 23 to Geddes Road. Turn right onto Geddes Road. Continue east on Geddes Road for approximately 0.1 mile; then turn left onto Dixboro Road. The gardens will be on your right after approximately 2 miles.

Matthaei Botanical Gardens: Fleming Creek, Marilyn Bland Prairie, and Sam Graham Trees Trails

SCENERY: ★ ★ ★
TRAIL CONDITION: ★ ★ ★
CHILDREN: ★ ★ ★
DIFFICULTY: ★ ★
SOLITUDE: ★ ★

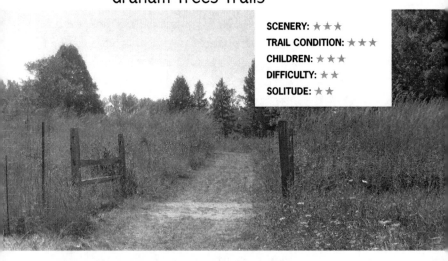

A TRAIL CUTS THROUGH A FIELD THICK WITH WILDFLOWERS.

GPS TRAILHEAD COORDINATES: N42° 17.991' W83° 39.651'

DISTANCE & CONFIGURATION: 1.3-mile loop

HIKING TIME: About 1 hour or less

HIGHLIGHTS: Woodlands, prairie, fields, Fleming Creek

ELEVATION: 790 feet at trailhead, with no significant rise

ACCESS: Daily, sunrise–sunset; no fees or permits required for grounds. Conservatory, garden shop, and visitor center: Monday, Tuesday, and Thursday–Sunday, 10 a.m.–4:30 p.m.; Wednesday, 10 a.m.–8 p.m. Adults, $5; children 5–18, $2; free, children under 5

MAPS: In the visitor center and at **mbgna.umich.edu**

FACILITIES: Conservatory, visitor center, garden shop, restrooms

WHEELCHAIR ACCESS: Yes, at the conservatory and display gardens, as well as the Sue Reichert Discovery Trail and the Sam Graham Trees Trail; no access at the Fleming Creek Trail

COMMENTS: Dogs are not permitted unless they are guide dogs. Bicycles are not allowed on the trails. The massasauga rattlesnake is frequently spotted on the grounds; give them plenty of space and do not touch.

CONTACTS: 734-647-7600; **mbgna.umich.edu**

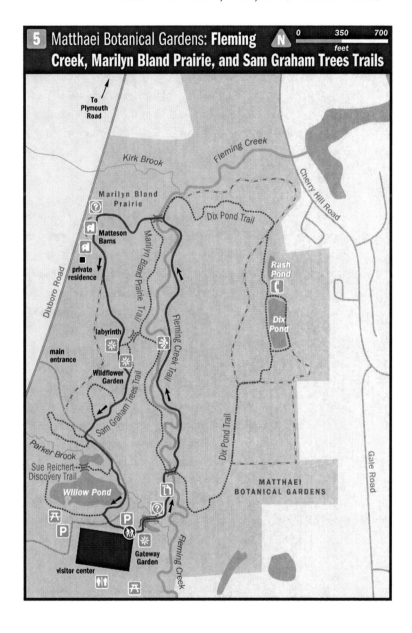

5 Matthaei Botanical Gardens: **Fleming Creek, Marilyn Bland Prairie, and Sam Graham Trees Trails**

0   350   700
feet

To Plymouth Road

Kirk Brook

Fleming Creek

Cherry Hill Road

Marilyn Bland Prairie

Dix Pond Trail

Matteson Barns

private residence

Marilyn Bland Prairie Trail

Dixboro Road

Rash Pond

Dix Pond

labyrinth

Fleming Creek Trail

main entrance

Wildflower Garden

Sam Graham Trees Trail

Dix Pond Trail

Gale Road

Parker Brook

Sue Reichert Discovery Trail

Willow Pond

MATTHAEI BOTANICAL GARDENS

visitor center

Gateway Garden

Fleming Creek

Overview

Combined, the Fleming Creek, Marilyn Bland Prairie, and Sam Graham Trees trails traverse all of the garden property's local habitats: floodplain, a small glacial hill, old woodlots, fallow fields, and a restored prairie. The Marilyn Bland Prairie Trail also crosses through the property of the Matteson barns and farmhouse along Dixboro Road.

Route Details

Begin at the trailhead located just beyond the Gateway Garden and reconstructed wetlands. Follow the wide stone path along a row of white cedars and across a 100-plus-foot-long wooden bridge (regard the sign on your right warning of TINY FROG CROSSING) that leads to a dirt gravel path. There, an earthen-roofed trail kiosk stands directly in front of you. This is the beginning of the Sam Graham Trees Trail that connects to the Fleming Creek Trail.

Beyond the kiosk, the wide dirt trail passes a variety of trees, including silver maples and tulip trees identified by small signs. At about the 0.2-mile mark, an observation deck overlooks Fleming Creek. A notable musclewood tree is identified on your left.

Cross a bridge to the opposite side of the creek, where the Fleming Creek Trail begins, and turn left (north). The Fleming Creek Trail traverses the eastern banks of the trail's namesake. Cottonwoods, walnut trees, burr oaks, and tamaracks dot the floodplain on both sides of the creek. Occasional paths lead through small openings down to the creek. These floodplain forests are here today because they were never lumbered; the land was too swampy. The American elms, larches, and ashes—dead but still standing—are victims of exotic invasive pests.

Continuing north, the trail rises slightly and becomes a grassy pathway high above the water. Just beyond the 0.5-mile mark, bear right along the flat trail. Around the 0.7-mile mark, the Fleming Creek Trail ends. Swing left, crossing the wooden bridge to the Marilyn

Bland Prairie Trail. After crossing the bridge, the dirt-gravel trail rises slightly and passes a big oak tree on your right. (Huge oak trees are common along the route.)

The trail leads to meadows or prairie openings, common before farming began in the area in the 1830s. The trail, grassy here, passes through the Marilyn Bland Prairie, the most diverse prairie on the property. Native Midwest plant species were planted here more than 50 years ago, and the tract served as an experimental research program for doctorate students at the University of Michigan. The prairie is a fire-maintained landscape, with burnings typically in the fall and spring.

After crossing the prairie, the trail swings south and passes a historical farmstead. This was the site of one of the earliest settlements in the Dixboro area. You can't miss the Matteson barns and farmhouse on your right; on your left, thick trees and shrubs border the trail and the west side of Fleming Creek. The trail becomes a dirt lane dividing fields and woods, passing under a big oak tree with branches hovering over the lane.

At about the 1-mile mark, the trail passes the Helen V. Smith Woodland Wildflower Garden on your left. Stone-lined dirt trails crisscross through woods, with small signs marking varieties of woodland wildflowers of the southern Great Lakes region. Depending on the time of year, you can see mayapples, twin leaf, wild leeks, Christmas ferns, wild sarsaparilla, cow parsnips, blue-eyed grass, and wild ginger, to name a few. Tree species also are identified, including black cherry trees, black oak trees, and quaking aspens.

At the wildflower garden, the Marilyn Bland Prairie Trail leads into the Sam Graham Trees Trail. At about the 1.1-mile mark, the trail veers away from the woods along a mowed trail. The fields are dotted with pines—and even rare blue spruces—and teeming with wildflowers. Dixboro Road is visible to the west. The trail crosses the road leading to the visitor center at about the 1.2-mile mark and ends at Willow and Park ponds.

Nearby Attractions

Head north on Dixboro Road and turn right onto Plymouth and you'll pass through the tiny village of Dixboro. On the north side of the street is the Dixboro General Store, long a landmark on the main road between Ann Arbor and Detroit. Built in 1840, the store over the years has sold a diverse mix of gasoline, general merchandise, and antiques—and once housed a local post office. Today, the store sells furniture, home accessories, candles, collectibles, and bath and body products.

Directions

From Detroit, take I-94 west to I-96, Exit 213B, toward Lansing. Follow it 18 miles and merge onto M-14 west, Exit 172, toward Ann Arbor. Continue on that highway for 12 miles to M-153 east, Exit 10. Turn right onto Plymouth–Ann Arbor Road and drive for 2 miles. Turn left onto North Dixboro Road. The gardens are about 1 mile down, on your left.

From Ann Arbor, take US 23 north for about 4.6 miles to Geddes Road, Exit 39. Turn right onto Geddes Road. Turn left onto North Dixboro Road. The gardens are 1.8 miles down, on your right.

University of Michigan Nichols Arboretum Trails

6

SCENERY: ★ ★ ★
TRAIL CONDITION: ★ ★ ★
CHILDREN: ★ ★ ★
DIFFICULTY: ★ ★
SOLITUDE: ★ ★

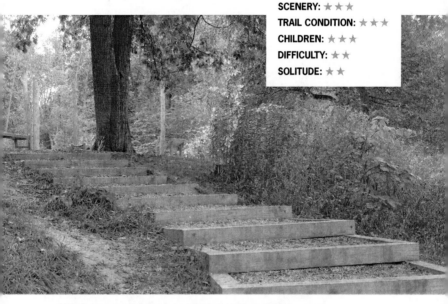

A SERIES OF STEPS LEADS DOWN TO THE SCENIC HURON RIVER.

GPS TRAILHEAD COORDINATES: N42° 16.843' W83° 43.610'

DISTANCE & CONFIGURATION: 3.4-mile connecting loops with a spur

HIKING TIME: About 1.5 hours

HIGHLIGHTS: Woodlands, fields, prairie, Huron River

ELEVATION: 868 at trailhead, with no significant rise

ACCESS: Daily, sunrise–sunset; no fees or permits required

MAPS: At information kiosks at Garden Gateway, Nichols Drive, and Geddes entrances and at **mbgna.umich.edu**

FACILITIES: Primitive restrooms along the trails. Public restrooms at the James D. Reader Jr. Center for Urban Environmental Education at the Washington Heights entrance.

WHEELCHAIR ACCESS: None

COMMENTS: Pets must be on leashes. Bikers are not permitted. Do not collect leaves, flowers, plants, or fruits. Paid parking is available within walking distance to the arboretum at city or University of Michigan health system parking lots. Free parking is available on the weekends at lot M-29 off East Medical Center Drive or lot M-28 on Washington Heights.

CONTACTS: 734-647-8986; **mbgna.umich.edu**

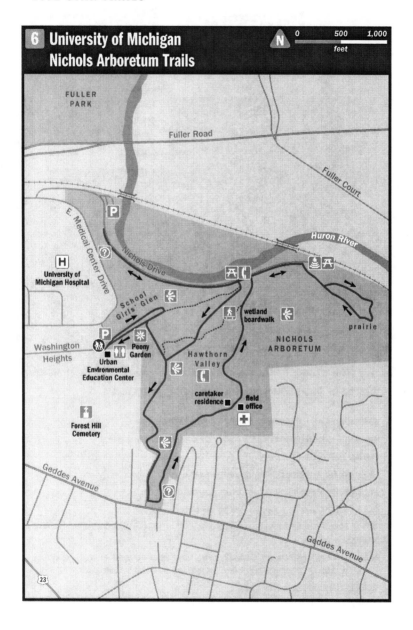

6 **University of Michigan Nichols Arboretum Trails**

N

0   500   1,000
feet

FULLER PARK

Fuller Road

Fuller Court

E. Medical Center Drive

P

Nichols Drive

Huron River

H
University of
Michigan Hospital

School Girls' Glen

wetland
boardwalk

prairie

NICHOLS
ARBORETUM

P

Washington
Heights

Peony
Garden

Urban
Environmental
Education Center

Hawthorn
Valley

caretaker
residence

field
office

Forest Hill
Cemetery

Geddes Avenue

Geddes Avenue

23

Overview

The network of trails at the Nichols Arboretum crisscross a diverse landscape of wooded hills, wetlands, shrub and flower gardens, prairies, and a long stretch of the Huron River. The Arb, as it's known locally, is a popular retreat for University of Michigan students, who come here to study, read, or sunbathe on grassy hillsides; picnic under majestic trees; or pursue a variety of outdoor activities, including running, disc sports, and hiking.

Route Details

The Nichols Arboretum is an urban oasis at the eastern edge of the University of Michigan central campus. It's long been a gathering spot for students, so hikers won't find much seclusion on the Arb's trails. Still, they're worth exploring for a variety of reasons, including the many gardens, second- and third-growth forests, and rare tree species.

What really makes the Arb so special is the design by O. C. Simonds, a landscape gardener who studied architecture at the University of Michigan. His 1906 design capitalizes on the views and celebrates the diverse topography with scenic hilltop and riverside overlooks, as well as a variety of tree and plant life. There is really no other park like the arboretum in the metropolitan region. And while the arboretum encompasses just 123 acres, the network of trails makes it feel much bigger.

The trails can be accessed from any of three entrances: Washington Heights, Geddes Road, and Nichols Drive, which borders the Huron River. Parking is available at both the Gateway and Nichols entrances. Information kiosks are posted at each entrance.

To follow the arboretum's trail sequence outlined on maps, begin at marker 1 at the Washington Heights entrance next to the

Urban Environmental Education Center at the Burnham House and Gateway Garden. This paved entrance opens up to a wide dirt trail that immediately passes the Burnham House and Peony Garden, both on the right. When in full bloom in late spring, the Peony Garden includes more than 10,000 flowers, and many of them are heirloom varieties from the 1800s and early 1900s.

Stay to the left of the Peony Garden as you head northeast en route to marker 2. On your left, you'll see School Girls' Glen, a steep, narrow valley that cuts northeast to the Huron River. In the spring, trilliums and other wildflowers bloom in the glen. Marker 2 stands at an intersection around the 0.2-mile mark. Swing right, heading south to marker 3.

This stretch of the trail borders an area known as the Heathdale, a cove of low-growing evergreen shrubs and plants common to the Appalachian Mountains. In the spring, a variety of azaleas, rhododendrons, and mountain laurels bloom in this secluded area.

Marker 3 is posted at 0.3 miles at an intersection of trails overlooking the Main Valley and arboretum. An overlook allows you to see how Simonds's design capitalized on the topography. At this juncture, continue straight, heading south. You'll pass a bench in a small clearing around the 0.5-mile mark. A sign notes a mature black walnut tree, cultivated in 1686.

The trail slopes slightly and reaches another overlook with a pair of cement benches at the 0.8-mile mark, near the Geddes entrance. Looking north from the overlook, you can see why the Main Valley is referred to as the hearth of the Arb, and you can again see how Simonds took advantage of the topography, retaining the slopes created from retreating glaciers more than 10,000 years ago.

Just ahead, at the Geddes entrance and marker 4, is the Centennial Shrub Collection, which features popular ornamental shrubs and small trees, including lilacs. From here, the trail loops north and northeast, reaching marker 5 around 1 mile.

You'll find marker 5 on your left as you come face to face with the arboretum's field office. Swing left along the wide dirt trail, passing the caretaker's home on your left. From here, the trail crosses through mostly open meadows scattered with trees, an area known as Hawthorn Valley.

Around the 1.4-mile mark, the trail comes to a T at the Riverfront Landing. Marker 7 is just to the left. To continue to marker 6, swing right, heading north-northeast along the riverfront, which is accessible by a series of steps. Marker 6 is at the 1.5-mile mark.

From here, hikers have their choice of continuing straight or east, as the trail parallels a railroad track and the Huron River, or swinging right directly toward the Alex Dow Prairie. Heading right or south toward the prairie, which is the route I took, the trail passes a picnic area and an amphitheater on the right. A series of trails cut through the Alex Dow field, part of an ongoing prairie restoration; controlled burns occur in the spring. Take a good look around for a glimpse of what this part of Michigan was like before large-scale settlement; most of the prairie species in the Alex Dow field have disappeared elsewhere in the region. Peak bloom time is in the summer, and big bluestem, the most common grass, peaks in early fall. Species blooming in the fall include yellow coneflowers, meadow roses, and black-eyed Susans. Doing a short loop through the prairie, initially cutting directly through the heart of the the prairie and then turning left at the first intersection, near the 1.8-mile mark, will add about 0.5 miles to your trip, returning you to marker 6 at the 2-mile mark. From marker 6, continue west along the river back toward marker 7, at that intersection of trails you came to previously. Marker 7 will be on your left at the 2.1-mile mark.

Continuing west, the trail parallels an open stretch of the Huron River, and marker 8 is at the 2.5-mile mark at the Nichols Drive entrance. Turn around and retrace your steps to marker 7. From there, bear right and continue south to marker 3, at the 3.1-mile mark. Follow the signposts back to the beginning point.

Nearby Attractions

Parker Mill County Park, about 5 miles away, is home to a historical gristmill, built in 1873 and open to public tours during fall weekends. The mostly wooded 26-acre park also is home to a mile-long board-walk, with signs identifying fauna and wildlife, along the end of Fleming Creek.

Directions

From Detroit, follow I-94 about 3 miles to I-96 west, Exit 213B to Lansing. Follow about 18 miles to Exit 45, M-14 west toward Ann Arbor. Exit at Geddes Road and follow east. Geddes turns into Fuller Road. Turn left on East Medical Center Drive and follow around the University of Michigan Hospital. Turn left on Observatory Street, then left on Washington Heights. The entrance is at the end of the street.

From Ann Arbor, follow US 23 to Exit 37B, Washtenaw Avenue. Follow Washtenaw Avenue west about 3 miles. Turn right on Observatory Street. Go about 0.3 miles and turn right on Washington Heights. The entrance is at the end of the street.

THE MARILYN BLAND PRAIRIE TRAIL PASSES BY A BARN.

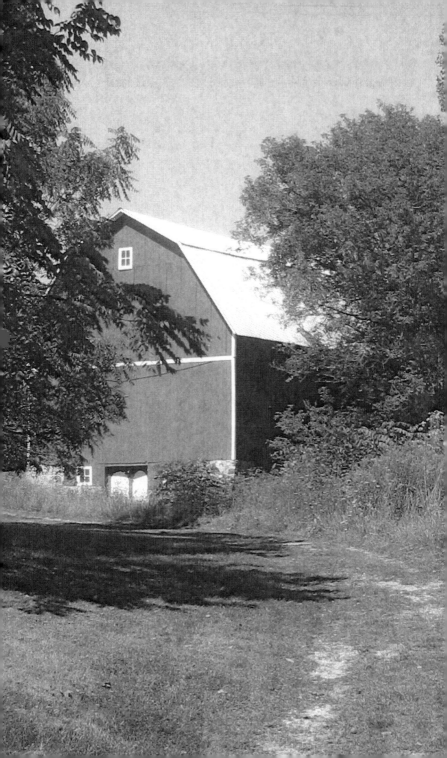

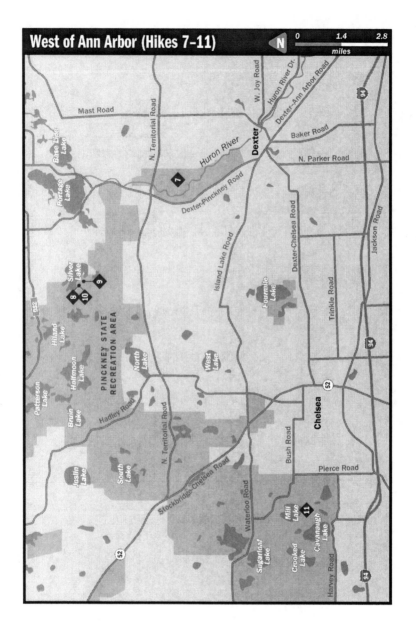

West of Ann Arbor (Hikes 7–11)

N

0   1.4   2.8
miles

West of Ann Arbor

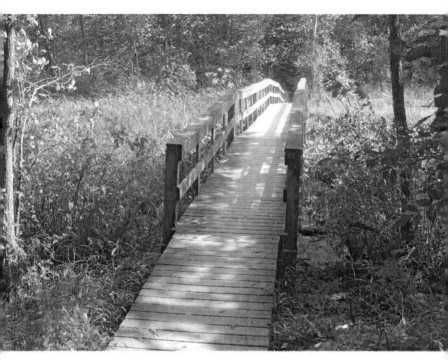

A BOARDWALK CROSSES THROUGH WETLANDS.

7

Hudson Mills Metropark:
Acorn Nature Trail

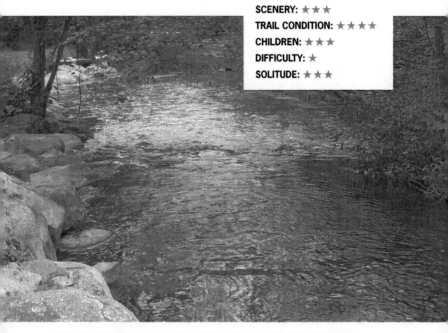

SCENERY: ★ ★ ★
TRAIL CONDITION: ★ ★ ★ ★
CHILDREN: ★ ★ ★
DIFFICULTY: ★
SOLITUDE: ★ ★ ★

A NARROW STRETCH OF THE HURON RIVER RIPPLES THROUGH THE PARK.

GPS TRAILHEAD COORDINATES: N42° 37.577' W83° 90.839'

DISTANCE & CONFIGURATION: 2-mile loop

HIKING TIME: About 1 hour or less

HIGHLIGHTS: Woodlands, Huron River

ELEVATION: 910 feet at trailhead, with no significant rise

ACCESS: April 2–October 31: Daily, 7 a.m.–10 p.m. November 1–April 1: Daily, 7 a.m.–8 p.m. Park office and activity center: Daily, 8 a.m.–4 p.m. $5 per vehicle per day or $25 per vehicle annually

MAPS: At the activity center or **metroparks.com**

FACILITIES: Restrooms, picnic areas, nature center

WHEELCHAIR ACCESS: None

COMMENTS: Pets, bicycles, and jogging are not permitted.

CONTACTS: 734-426-8211; **metroparks.com**

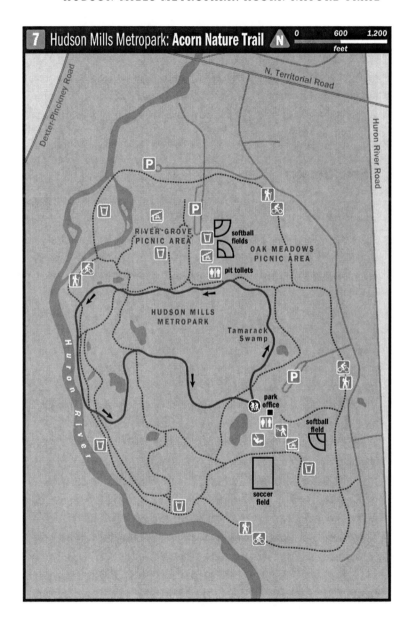

Overview

The Acorn Nature Trail weaves through woods, a tamarack swamp, and along the banks of a scenic stretch of the Huron River frequented by kayakers and canoeists. The landscape of woods, fields, and swamps is especially beautiful in the fall with maples, oaks, and hardwoods exploding in brilliant colors.

Route Details

Hudson Mills Metropark derives its name from three mills that once stood along the banks of the Huron River, not far from the present-day site of the Hudson Mills Metropark Activity Center. The first of the three mills, a gristmill, was built in the 1840s. Known as Hudson Mill, the gristmill processed flour and corn and eventually produced 6,000 barrels of flour a year.

A cider mill and a plaster mill followed, and the settlement became known as Hudson Mills. The community included a handful of homes, a school, a hotel, and a cemetery. Today, all that remains of the actual mills are their stone foundations. They are visible at the northern neck of the park near the river at the aptly named Rapids View Picnic Area, and they can be seen from a spur off the Hike-Bike Trail, just beyond the River Grove Picnic Area.

Little else remains to remind hikers of Hudson Mills's past, although exhibits in the activity center display historical photographs of the mills and include a gristmill stone. Even so, the 1,549-acre park boasts a wealth of amenities. In addition to coming here for the park's two major hiking trails—the Acorn Nature Trail and the paved Hike-Bike Trail—outdoor enthusiasts enjoy canoeing, an 18-hole golf course, disc golf, and a variety of sports fields.

The Acorn Nature Trail, as the name implies, is the more rustic of the two paths. Beyond the experience of walking through maturing hardwoods, this nature trail offers hikers up-close views of a tamarack swamp and a scenic stretch of the winding Huron River.

You will begin the Acorn Nature Trail just outside the activity center, past a grassy picnic area. There's no trailhead per se, just a wooden sign that reads NATURE TRAIL. Another sign, just to the left, reads ACORN TRAIL. They are one and the same, the beginning and the end of the 2-mile trail that winds northwest of the activity center. Hikers can go in either direction.

Most hikers choose to bear right, following the Nature Trail, a wide dirt path that immediately passes a small amphitheater used for nature-related programs. The footpath slopes slightly and crosses a park service drive. From there, continue straight along the path following a small wooden sign that reads ACORN NATURE TRAIL.

The trail almost immediately crosses a tamarack swamp, an expansive marsh littered with dead trees and framed by poison sumacs and red osier dogwoods. The ubiquitous tamarack, an unusual conifer that loses its needles in the fall, towers above the marshland. In the fall, their green needles turn golden before they drop, and the tree looks deceptively dead until spring.

The trail is a mix of gravel and dirt as it veers through woodlands. The only man-made intrusions are occasional benches and small interpretive signs explaining various habitats, including meadows frequented by white-tailed deer and river life.

At about 0.5 miles into the woods, the trail begins to veer away from the tamarack swamp and passes a vegetation enclosure plot, a small patch of woods and brush being studied to determine the impact of white-tailed deer on the surrounding landscape.

Most of the trail remains deep in the woods, occasionally intersecting the paved Hike-Bike Trail and paralleling the metropark's service drive for a stretch.

At about 0.8 miles, the trail parallels the shoreline of the Huron River, just below the rapids at the northern end of the park. This stretch of the winding river attracts canoeists, fishermen, and picnickers. Thus, picnic tables and grills dot the eastern shoreline.

The trail eventually meanders back through the woods, crosses a wooden bridge over a small stream, and passes emerald ash borer traps—small trees with blue signs posted on them. Veer right at the sign for NATURE TRAIL and continue along the wide dirt path as it passes through an edge, the spot where two different habitats meet. Follow the trail back to the activity center.

Nearby Attractions

Thickly wooded, the nearby Dexter-Huron Metropark, about 5 miles away, is an ideal spot for a picnic. The 122-acre landscape borders the Huron River, just 7.5 miles northwest of Ann Arbor. It also features a canoe launch, playground, and softball field. You will often see fishermen along this stretch of the river.

Directions

From Detroit, follow the Lodge Freeway north to I-94 west, Exit 4B. Merge onto I-96 westbound, Exit 213B, toward Lansing. Continue 18.4 miles to M-14 west toward Ann Arbor. Follow M-14 for 17.4 miles to US 23 north toward Brighton and Flint. Take Exit 49, Territorial Road. Turn left on East North Territorial Road. As this road heads westward to Hudson Mills Metropark, its name changes slightly along the way. After 0.3 miles, the road becomes North Territorial Road West; follow it for 2.2 miles. Then it turns into West North Territorial Road; follow that for 1 mile. Finally, the road becomes North Territorial Road. Follow that west about 4.5 miles to the park entrance, which will be on the south side of the road.

From Ann Arbor, take US 23 north to Exit 49, Territorial Road. Turn left on East North Territorial Road. As this road heads westward to the park, its name changes slightly along the way. After 0.3 miles, the road becomes North Territorial Road West; follow that for 2.2 miles. When it turns into West North Territorial Road, follow that for 1 mile. Finally, the road becomes North Territorial Road. Follow that west for about 4.5 miles to the park entrance, which will be on the south side of the road.

8

Pinckney State Recreation Area:
Crooked Lake Trail

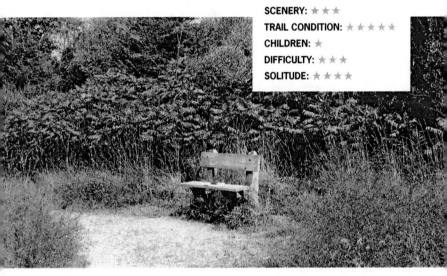

SCENERY: ★ ★ ★
TRAIL CONDITION: ★ ★ ★ ★ ★
CHILDREN: ★
DIFFICULTY: ★ ★ ★
SOLITUDE: ★ ★ ★ ★

A BENCH INVITES HIKERS TO STOP AND ENJOY A VIEW OF CROOKED LAKE.

GPS TRAILHEAD COORDINATES: N42° 41.732' W83° 96.413'

DISTANCE & CONFIGURATION: 5.1-mile loop

HIKING TIME: About 2 hours

HIGHLIGHTS: Woodlands, wetlands, Crooked Lake, Pickerel Lake

ELEVATION: 880 feet at trailhead; 1,008 feet at highest point

ACCESS: Daily, 8 a.m.–10 p.m.; $10 annual recreation passport per vehicle

MAPS: At the park office on Silver Hill Road or **michigan.gov/dnr**

FACILITIES: Restrooms, picnic area, beach

WHEELCHAIR ACCESS: None

COMMENTS: Trail passes through area open to hunting in season. Trail is open to mountain bikers. Bikers are required to travel in a clockwise direction; hikers are asked to head in the opposite direction, counterclockwise. The weekends are especially busy with bikers.

CONTACTS: 734-426-4913; **michigan.gov/dnr**

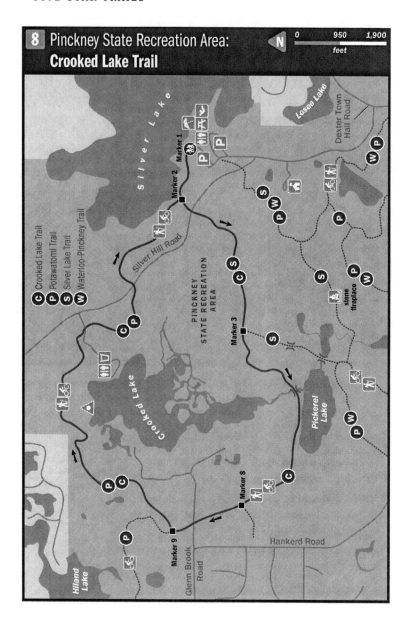

Overview

The longest of the day-hiking trails within the boundaries of Pinckney State Recreation Area, Crooked Lake winds deep into hardwood forests; over rolling, sometimes rugged terrain; and by lakes and wetlands. The trail rarely leaves the forest and is especially beautiful in October when the oaks, maples, and other trees are turning colors. This is one of the premier hiking trails in southeast Michigan.

Route Details

The Pinckney State Recreation Area straddles Livingston and Washtenaw counties, and its rugged terrain offers some of the most scenic hiking in southeastern Michigan. The 11,000-acre park is well known among mountain bikers for its challenging routes, particularly the Potawatomi Trail, also known as "the Hills of Hell." The state recreation area is a sprawling swath of forests, lakes, and wetlands. Consisting largely of reclaimed farmland, the park is home to second-growth forests—woods that have been wild long enough to offer a sense of backcountry. Few traces of the farmers and mill operators who once worked this land remain.

Both the Crooked Lake and Silver Lake trailheads are located just off the northwest corner of the upper parking lot in the day-use area at Silver Lake. Bikers begin in the southwest corner, at marker

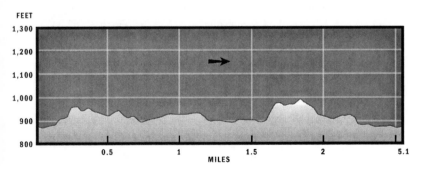

7, the end of the Silver Lake Trail, so that bikers and hikers travel in opposite directions and are clearly visible to one another.

The trailhead for hikers, at marker 1, is about 100 feet off the *northwest corner* of the upper parking lot near the picnic area at Silver Lake. You'll see picnic tables and grills, a concession stand, and beach house at the edge of the parking lot. Swing left from the parking area, walking through the grassy area to the trailhead.

The trail dips immediately into the woods, and along this short stretch—just 0.2 miles—you'll mostly walk with Silver Lake on one side and wetlands on the other. The lake is often visible through the trees. It's a prime location to see waterfowl in the spring and fall. Wildflowers are abundant in those seasons as well.

At marker 2, continue straight, heading northwest to marker 9, a little more than 2 miles away. The natural inclination is to swing left and head to marker 3, but for the safety of hikers, park officials recommend continuing in a counterclockwise direction. This is the longest stretch between markers and the trail stays mostly under the cover of a forest of black, red, and white oaks, as well as hickory and maple trees. The lake and the wetlands buffering its western edges remain visible through the trees. The trail rises and dips, with occasional rocky slopes.

After crossing Silver Hill Road, around the 1-mile mark, the trail winds along the crest of a hill, with steep ravines on either side. The trail again crosses Silver Hill Road and becomes more rugged, with elevation rising above 1,000 feet. An overlook of sorts—a clearing with a bench—is at the 1.2-mile mark. The bench is situated so hikers can rest and look southwest to Crooked Lake and the forested ridges beyond, but when the foliage is thick, there is little to see.

The trail gradually descends to a small wooden bridge crossing a creek connecting Crooked and Hiland lakes (neither is visible at this point). You can glimpse Crooked Lake through the trees around the 1.5-mile mark. The trail becomes gentler, angling southwest through more marshlands, and reaches marker 9 at 2.4 miles.

Marker 9 also is a junction with the Potawatomi Trail, which heads off in a northwesterly direction. Continue straight, heading south and crossing Glenbrook Road. The trail flattens but continues through the woods on the opposite side of the road. Don't be surprised to hear the sounds of cars and trucks as you walk this stretch close to Hankerd Road. From marker 9, you begin to loop back to the trailhead.

The trees create a canopy effect as you approach marker 8, which stands ahead in a small clearing. A spur on your right leads to Hankerd Road and a parking lot on the opposite side. Void of much of the shrubbery and brush that dots the forest, the trail immediately passes through a lengthy stand of towering maple trees. Pickerel Lake comes into view as the stand of maples thins. The trail rises above the lake, offering scenics of the undeveloped lake. Around the 3.6-mile mark, the trail drops to a boardwalk crossing a thick wetlands and stream running between Crooked and Pickerel lakes.

Heading northeast, the trail climbs more hills and reaches marker 3 at 3.9 miles. Because the Crooked Lake and Silver Lake trails diverge for about a mile, the trail markers are out of sequence on the Crooked Lake Trail. Marker 3 stands at the junction of the Crooked Lake and Silver Lake trails. Go straight, heading due east toward marker 2. The trail rises again, climbing above swamps on either side to an elevation of 970 feet. The trail again crosses Silver Hill Road before returning to marker 2. Turn right and retrace your steps to marker 1 and the trailhead at the northeast corner of the upper parking lot.

Nearby Attractions

One of the youngest metroparks, Huron Meadows Metropark is about 16 miles northeast of the Pinckney State Recreation Area, near Brighton. The 1,566-acre park boasts an 18-hole golf course and Maltby Lake, open to swimmers, boaters, and anglers. Picnic areas overlook the lake. The park's most notable trail loops around the lake, through woods and rolling meadows.

Directions

From Detroit, take I-94 west about 3 miles to I-96 west to Lansing, Exit 213B. Go about 18 miles and merge left onto M-14 to Ann Arbor (crossing under I-275). Go another 18 miles and merge onto US 23 north to Brighton/Flint and take Exit 49, North Territorial Road. Turn left on North Territorial and follow it about 11 miles to Dexter Town Hall Road. Turn right. Continue about 1 mile and turn left onto Silver Hill Road, where you will see the park entrance.

From Ann Arbor, take US 23 north to Exit 49, North Territorial Road. Turn left and continue about 11 miles to Dexter Town Hall Road. Turn right. Go another 1 mile and turn left onto Silver Hill Road, where you will see the park entrance.

9

Pinckney State Recreation Area:
Losee Lake Trail

SCENERY: ★ ★ ★
TRAIL CONDITION: ★ ★
CHILDREN: ★
DIFFICULTY: ★ ★
SOLITUDE: ★ ★ ★

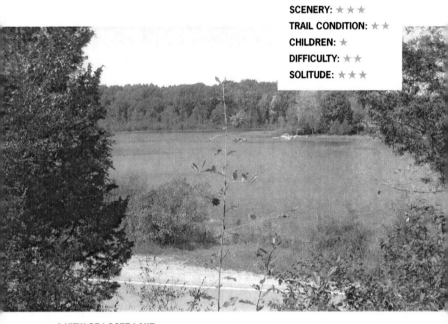

A VIEW OF LOSEE LAKE

GPS TRAILHEAD COORDINATES: N42° 41.561' W83° 96.272'

DISTANCE & CONFIGURATION: 3.3-mile loop

HIKING TIME: About 2 hours

HIGHLIGHTS: Woodlands, wetlands, Losee Lake

ELEVATION: 860 feet at trailhead, with no significant rise

ACCESS: Daily, 8 a.m.–10 p.m.; $10 annual recreation passport per vehicle

MAPS: At the park office on Silver Hill Road or **michigan.gov/dnr**

FACILITIES: Restrooms, picnic area, playground, beach

WHEELCHAIR ACCESS: None

COMMENTS: Pets must be on leashes. No bikes allowed on this trail.

CONTACTS: 734-426-4913; **michigan.gov/dnr**

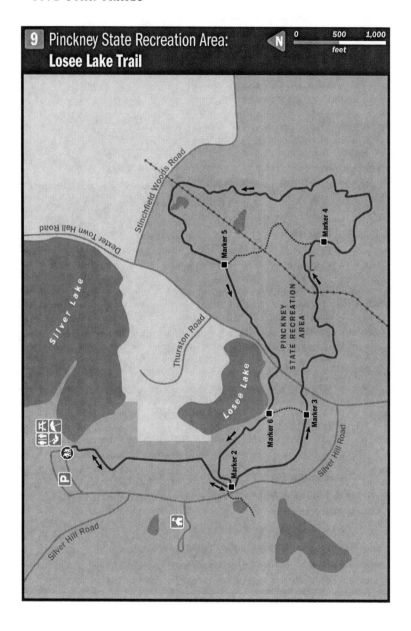

Overview

Despite its name, the Losee Lake Trail spends little time around its namesake lake, though there are some nice views of the water along the last stretch of the hike. The trail covers ground similar to the longer Crooked Lake Trail and rarely ventures outside the forest cover. The grassy picnic area at the trailhead belies some of the rugged terrain along its route.

Route Details

Most of the Losee Lake Trail rambles through woods dotted with wetlands and ponds. Hikers will enjoy glimpses of Losee Lake at the trailhead and then again as the trail winds back to its beginning. The trail is actually a series of three connecting loops, the first beginning about 0.5 miles from the trailhead. Follow the shortest loop for a 1.5-mile hike, the middle loop for a 2.5-mile hike, or the longest, for 3.3 miles. This description encompasses the longest route. Like the other trails at the Pinckney State Recreation Area, the Losee Lake Trail is well marked, using Michigan's state trail-marker system, with markers typically placed at trail intersections.

The trailhead is located about 50 feet southeast of the lower parking lot at the Silver Lake day-use area. Standing at the trailhead, you'll see a grill and a pair of picnic tables under an oak tree nearby. Losee Lake lies right in front of you as well. Follow the grassy swath past the picnic area, and at about 450 feet, swing right up a hill, past a bench beneath an apple tree, and head into the woods. You're heading to marker 2.

The trail narrows as it slips into the woods, and any glimpses of the lake disappear. The landscape along this stretch is similar to what hikers will encounter along much of the route: rolling woodlands, occasional wetlands crossed by boardwalks, ponds, and steep ravines. An impressive stand of towering pines lines a portion of the trail en route to marker 2. Be aware that a grassy trail veering off on the left at a split-rail fence is private property. Continue straight past the fence. The trail takes a steep drop as it approaches marker 2, around the 0.5-mile mark.

Continue straight at marker 2, heading southeast to marker 3; this is part of the shortest of the three connecting loops. Boardwalks guide hikers through wetlands, teeming with wildflowers in the spring and fall. Marker 3 stands around the 0.7-mile point. This intersection affords a shortcut to marker 6. Continue straight to marker 4, heading southeast and along a boardwalk before crossing Dexter Town Hall Road.

Before reaching marker 4, the trail leaves the woods, crossing through a field and under power lines. Marker 4 stands in a clearing around the 1-mile point at the junction of the outer link of the middle loop. Swing right, past a bench on your left, heading southeast. This is the longest stretch between markers along the trail: it's about 1 mile to marker 5. The trail slopes and winds through the woods and across boardwalks through wetlands. The trail then swings north-northwest and up a steep hill, rising about 100 feet. A bench at the top of the hill makes a good stopping point if you need a rest. For a long stretch the trail passes an area free of the forest canopy, and the shrubbery and brush become so thick in spots that they create a wall-like effect. The trail crosses back through the field with the power lines before reaching marker 5.

At marker 5, continue straight (southwest) to marker 6, less than 0.5 miles ahead. An expansive wetland becomes visible through the trees on your left as you head southwest. You'll catch glimpses of Losee Lake just before the trail crosses Dexter Town Hall Road, and you can see a house across the lake. Marker 6 stands at around 2.4 miles. Head straight to marker 2. A sign points the way to the Silver Lake parking lot. A long boardwalk zigzags through wetlands, and you'll see the lake on your right.

At marker 2, climb up the hill and swing right, heading back to the trailhead. Another sign notes the direction to the Silver Lake parking lot.

Nearby Attractions

The region abounds with state, metro, and county parks. Independence Lake County Park, about 12.5 miles away, offers a variety of outdoor recreation, including hiking, swimming, boating, fishing, and picnicking. The Washtenaw County park's hiking trails crisscross wetlands, prairies, woods, and an impressive stand of oaks. A paved multiuse trail also runs through the park.

Directions

From Detroit, take I-94 west about 3 miles to I-96 west to Lansing, Exit 213B. Go about 18 miles and merge left onto M-14 to Ann Arbor (crossing under I-275). Go another 18 miles and merge onto US 23 north to Brighton/Flint. Take Exit 49, North Territorial Road. Turn left on North Territorial and follow it about 11 miles to Dexter Town Hall Road. Turn right. Continue about 1 mile and turn left onto Silver Hill Road, where you will see the park entrance.

From Ann Arbor, take US 23 north to Exit 49, North Territorial Road. Turn left and follow it about 11 miles to Dexter Town Hall Road. Turn right. Go 1 mile and turn left onto Silver Hill Road and into the park entrance.

10

Pinckney State Recreation Area:

Silver Lake Trail

SCENERY: ★ ★ ★
TRAIL CONDITION: ★ ★ ★ ★ ★
CHILDREN: ★ ★ ★
DIFFICULTY: ★ ★
SOLITUDE: ★ ★ ★

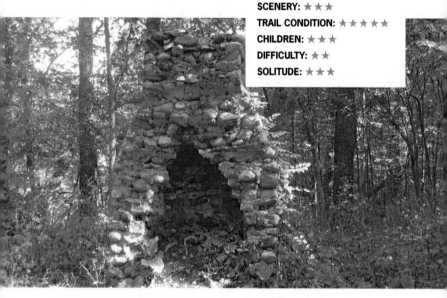

A STONE FIREPLACE STANDS AS A REMINDER OF HUMAN SETTLEMENT.

GPS TRAILHEAD COORDINATES: N42° 41.732' W83° 96.413'

DISTANCE & CONFIGURATION: 1.9-mile loop

HIKING TIME: About 1 hour or less

HIGHLIGHTS: Silver Lake, woods, wetlands

ELEVATION: 880 feet at trailhead; 970 feet at highest point

ACCESS: Daily, 8 a.m.–10 p.m.; $10 annual recreation passport per vehicle

MAPS: At the park office on Silver Hill Road or **michigan.gov/dnr**

FACILITIES: Restrooms, picnic area, playground, beach

WHEELCHAIR ACCESS: None

COMMENTS: Portions of the trail are shared with bikers, who are required to travel clockwise. Hikers are encouraged to walk counterclockwise.

CONTACTS: 734-426-4913; **michigan.gov/dnr**

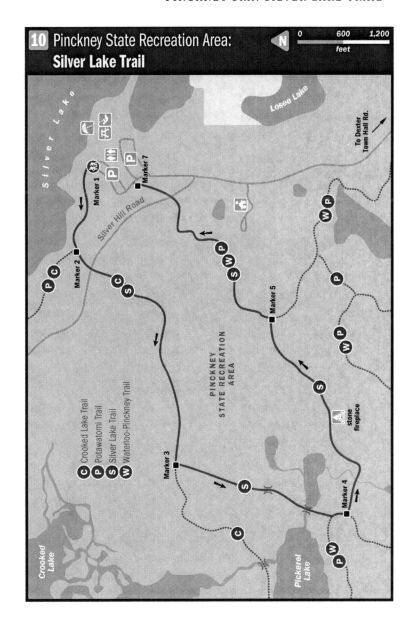

10 Pinckney State Recreation Area:
Silver Lake Trail

N

0   600   1,200
feet

Loseo Lake

To Dexter
Town Hall Rd.

Silver Lake

Marker 1

Marker 7

Silver Hill Road

P

P

W P

P

S W

Marker 2

P C

C

S

Marker 5

W P

S

PINCKNEY
STATE RECREATION
AREA

stone
fireplace

S

C Crooked Lake Trail
P Potawatomi Trail
S Silver Lake Trail
W Waterloo-Pinckney Trail

Marker 3

S

Marker 4

W

P

Crooked
Lake

Pickerel
Lake

Overview

The shortest of Pinckney State Recreation Area's hiking trails, the 1.9-mile Silver Lake Trail begins along the shores of Silver Lake but almost immediately veers westward through hardwood forests and wetlands. The terrain is moderately hilly, and the landscape is reminiscent of northern Michigan's backcountry.

Route Details

One of the largest state parks in southeast Michigan, the 11,000-acre Pinckney State Recreation Area is well liked by hikers, backpackers, mountain bikers, and anglers. Among the many parks that dot the southeastern Michigan landscape, Pinckney comes closest to replicating the backcountry of the upper Lower Peninsula. It's also home to two notable trails—the 17-mile Potawatomi Trail, contained entirely in the park and open to hikers, bikers, and cross-country skiers, and the 35-mile Pinckney-Waterloo Trail, which runs west to the much larger Waterloo State Recreation Area.

The trailhead for both the Silver Lake and Crooked Lake trails is located off the northwest corner of the upper parking lot in the day-use area at Silver Lake. Swing left off the edge of the parking lot closest to the lake, past a grassy picnic area, and you'll find the trailhead about 100 feet away. This is marker 1. Bikers are required to begin at marker 7, off the southwestern corner of the parking lot.

The trail immediately descends into the woods, skirting along the shores of Silver Lake. Brush is thick on either side, and although the wetlands on your left seem calm, listen closely and you'll likely hear plenty of aquatic life. For a short stretch, the trail runs between the lake and wetlands, a prime area for waterfowl sightings in the spring and fall.

At marker 2, just 0.2 miles from the trailhead, the trail swings south and then west, ambling away from the lake and deep into the forest of hickory and white, red, and black oaks. The Silver Lake and Crooked Lake trails continue to be one and the same along this stretch; note, however, that a portion of the Crooked Lake Trail continues straight or in a northwesterly direction at marker 2. After crossing Silver Hill Road, the terrain becomes quite hilly, rising to nearly 1,000 feet, and passes along the crests of hills with ravines on both sides and swamp visible below.

At marker 3, the Crooked Lake and Silver Lake trails diverge. Swing left, heading southwest to continue on the Silver Lake Trail. The trail becomes flatter along this stretch, passing through more wetlands. They are thick with brush and felled and dead trees and, in season, abloom with wildflowers along the banks.

Before reaching marker 4, you will come to a boardwalk that crosses the wetlands between Pickerel Lake on the right (west) side and a smaller lake on the opposite. It's a great spot to stop and take pictures or enjoy the views of the lake, where kayakers gather in the warmer months. Swing left at the intersection, continuing in an easterly direction toward marker 4, which is just ahead.

The trail slopes downward and crosses a bridge over a small creek that connects two small lakes. Lots of pines crowd the shorelines of the lake on your left. You'll pass large oak trees, a stone fireplace, and a bench as you head to marker 5. The terrain becomes hillier, with ravines on either side. At marker 5, continue in the same direction to marker 7, the end of the trail. Heading southeast to marker 6 leads to the Potawatomi Trail. The Silver Lake Trail ends at marker 7 in the lower parking lot of the day-use area.

Nearby Attractions

About 5 miles west on North Territorial Road, Park Lyndon County Park is home to 2 miles of marked trails that meander through sometimes-steep hillsides and a wetland community of oaks, hickory, and tamaracks. Ten species of orchids and more than 23 fern species flourish under the forest canopy. A portion of the trail runs across a long winding ridge, an unusual glacial landform created by ancient streams. The 335-acre park is part of the Washtenaw County park system.

Directions

From Detroit, take I-94 west about 3 miles to I-96 west to Lansing, Exit 213B. Go about 18 miles and merge left onto M-14 to Ann Arbor (crossing under I-275). In another 18 miles, merge onto US 23 north to Brighton/Flint. Take Exit 49, North Territorial Road. Turn left on North Territorial and follow it about 11 miles to Dexter Town Hall Road. Turn right. Continue about 1 mile and turn left onto Silver Hill Road and into the park entrance.

From Ann Arbor, take US 23 north to Exit 49, North Territorial Road. Turn left and follow it about 11 miles to Dexter Town Hall Road. Turn right. Go another 1 mile and turn left onto Silver Hill Road and into the park entrance.

11

Waterloo State Recreation Area:

Hickory Hills Trail

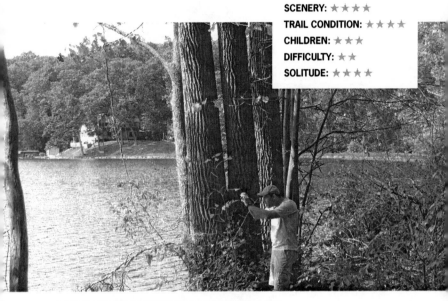

SCENERY: ★ ★ ★ ★
TRAIL CONDITION: ★ ★ ★ ★
CHILDREN: ★ ★ ★
DIFFICULTY: ★ ★
SOLITUDE: ★ ★ ★ ★

A HIKER SHOOTS PHOTOGRAPHS OF CROOKED LAKE.

GPS TRAILHEAD COORDINATES: N42° 19.320' W84° 5.230'

DISTANCE & CONFIGURATION: 5.3-mile balloon

HIKING TIME: About 3 hours

HIGHLIGHTS: Woodlands, wetlands, lakes

ELEVATION: 1,010 at trailhead; 1,091 feet at highest point

ACCESS: Daily, 8 a.m.–10 p.m.; $10 annual recreation passport per vehicle. Gerald E. Eddy Discovery Center: Open the week after Easter until the Sunday before Thanksgiving: Tuesday–Saturday, 10 a.m.–5 p.m.; Sunday, noon–5 p.m.

MAPS: At the Gerald E. Eddy Discovery Center or **michigan.gov/dnr**

FACILITIES: Gerald E. Eddy Discovery Center, restrooms, picnic pavilion, observation deck

WHEELCHAIR ACCESS: Yes, at the discovery center but not on the trail

COMMENTS: Sections of the Hickory Hills Trail pass through areas open to hunting.

CONTACTS: 734-475-3170; **michigan.gov/dnr**

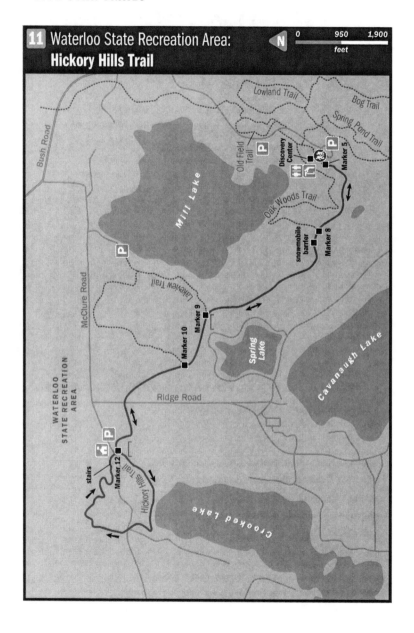

Overview

The longest of the Gerald E. Eddy Discovery Center trails, the aptly named Hickory Hills Trail passes through oak-hickory forests and remnants of an old golf course. The trail also covers some of the hilliest terrain in the state park and passes scenic Crooked Lake (a different lake from the one of the same name at Pinckney State Recreation Area). The balloon at the end of the trail serves as a nature trail. Its interpretive signs note varying aspects of the forest, including remnants of a domestic apple orchard, a dry marsh that was once a glacial lake, and current wildlife.

Route Details

The seven trails outside the Gerald R. Eddy Discovery Center manage to traverse only a small section of the more than 20,000-acre Waterloo State Recreation Area, the largest state recreation area in Michigan's Lower Peninsula. The Hickory Hills Trail is the longest of the seven. The others range from the 0.8-mile Old Field Trail to the 3.6-mile Lakeview Trail. The latter intersects with the Hickory Hills Trail and derives its name from its views of Mill Lake. All the trails begin in and around the parking lot outside the discovery center.

The trailhead for Hickory Hills is several feet off the western edge of the parking lot outside the discovery center. You'll see the

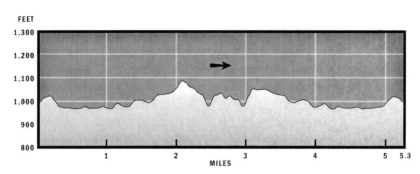

familiar Michigan state system's trail map at marker 5. Follow the narrow dirt trail as it winds through the woods in a southwesterly direction to marker 6. The oak and hickory forests here are thick, and you'll notice a ravine on your right as the trail slopes and becomes rocky. The trail passes Spring Pond and a bench on your left around the 0.3-mile mark.

The trail flattens and intersects with marker 8 and the Oak Woods Trail about 0.1 mile farther. The Oak Woods Trail stretches 1.3 miles off on the right, crossing a ridge through the oak-hickory forest and eventually running parallel to Mill Lake. To stay on the Hickory Hills Trail, continue straight, heading northwest. The trail passes through a snowmobile barrier before wetlands frame both sides of the trail. The stretch remains thick with woods and brush on either side.

Around the 0.7-mile mark, an earthen bridge crosses over a creek and the trail passes through more wetlands. The trail rises and dips through the woods, reaching an intersection with the Lakeview Trail around the 1-mile mark, or marker 9. You'll notice a bench on your left. This stretch of the Hickory Hills Trail also serves as the southern end of the Lakeview Trail loop. Continue straight or in a northwesterly direction.

After crossing through a small clearing, the trail dips back into the woods, passing wetlands and a house. Beyond the house you can see Spring Lake. You should reach marker 10 around the 1.1-mile mark. At 0.2 miles later, the trail forks around a large rock smack in the middle. You'll notice a metal fence on the right. A sign posted here also cautions that this part of the trail passes through areas open to hunting. While donning an orange vest or other appropriate gear is recommended, my advice is to avoid areas open to hiking during hunting season.

The trail crosses Ridge Road, and around the 1.5-mile mark, the trail empties into a grassy area outside the park headquarters, a brick ranch house with a flagpole in front. In the clearing, on the south side of McClure Road, you'll find marker 12 and a pair of benches underneath a cluster of trees. Continue straight (west) to marker 13, following a grassy swath back in the woods. This portion of the trail also serves as a nature trail; you'll notice signs marking everything from wildlife to the life cycle of the forest. The trail slopes gradually as it reaches Crooked Lake, which was formed by receding glaciers some 10,000 years ago. The lake becomes visible around the 1.7-mile mark and the trail drops another 100 feet before it reaches the shoreline. A perfectly positioned bench offers a panoramic view of the lake.

The trail follows the shoreline for a short stretch but then rises almost 150 feet to an overlook with a bench. Around the 2-mile mark, the trail descends slightly with a set of man-made stairs helping hikers down to McClure Road, the same road the park headquarters is located on, just to the east. Swing left, heading north-northwest; the trail becomes visible in the woods. The trail climbs slightly to marker 13. Continue straight (an arrow on the signpost will point you back to marker 12, the direction from which you came). You're continuing along the northern edge of the loop or nature trail.

You'll step down another set of man-made stairs and pass wetlands and a swampy stretch before the trail starts to climb again, as much as 100 feet. The trail returns to park headquarters near the 2.6-mile mark. Cross McClure Road and head back to marker 12. From there, head south-southeast back into the woods, retracing your route to the discovery center.

At the discovery center, an outside observation deck offers a broad view of Mill Lake to the northwest. Inside, exhibits, maps, and habitat dioramas explain the area's natural and human history. There's also a display of Native American artifacts and a hands-on area for children.

Nearby Attractions

One of the region's most well-known long-distance trails, the Waterloo-Pinckney Hiking Trail begins in and crosses through much of the Waterloo State Recreation Area. The trail stretches from

Big Portage Lake in Waterloo's western edge to Silver Lake in the Pinckney State Recreation Area, about 36 miles northeast. Along the way, the trails cut through oak-pine forests, glacial features (including kettle lakes), swamps, and abandoned farm fields. Campsites along the way allow ample shelter for backpacking trips lasting as long as four days.

Directions

From Detroit, take I-94 east about 3 miles to I-96 west to Lansing. Continue west about 19 miles. Take Exit 45, M-14, left toward Ann Arbor. Follow that about 5 miles and merge onto I-94 west. Continue about 14 miles to Exit 157, Pierce Road. Turn right and go north about 2.4 miles to Bush Road. Turn left and continue west, following the signs to Waterloo State Recreation Area and the discovery center.

From Ann Arbor, take I-94 east to Exit 157, Pierce Road. Turn right and follow Pierce Road north about 2.4 miles to Bush Road. Turn left and follow the signs to the Waterloo State Recreation Area and the discovery center.

THE TRAIL NARROWS THROUGH THICK WOODS.

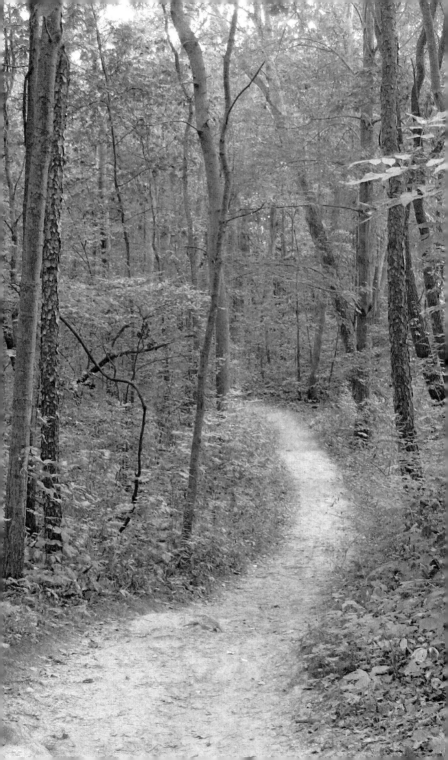

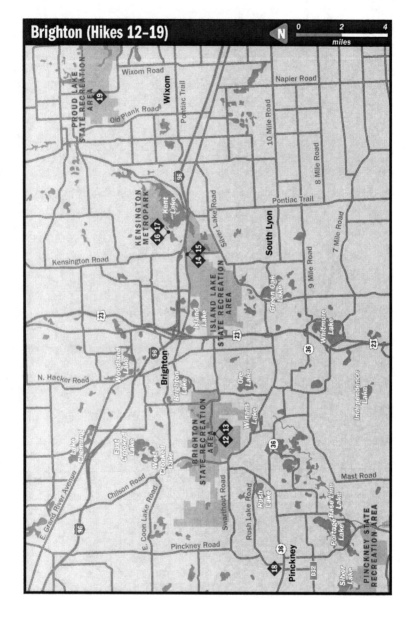

Brighton

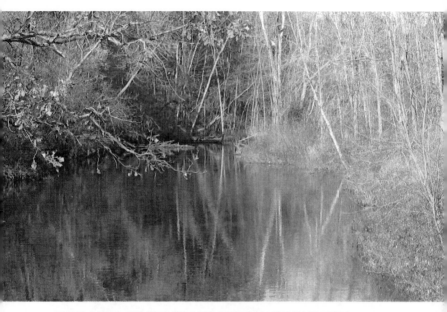

RIVERS, PONDS, AND WETLANDS ARE COMMON ALONG MOST TRAILS.

12

Brighton State Recreation Area:

Kahchin Trail

SCENERY: ★ ★
TRAIL CONDITION: ★ ★ ★ ★
CHILDREN: ★ ★ ★
DIFFICULTY: ★ ★
SOLITUDE: ★ ★ ★ ★

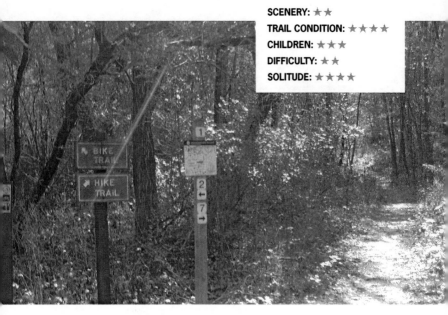

SIGNS POINT THE WAY FOR HIKERS AND BIKERS.

GPS TRAILHEAD COORDINATES: N42° 50.072' W83° 83.466'
DISTANCE & CONFIGURATION: 2-mile loop
HIKING TIME: About 1 hour
HIGHLIGHTS: Woods, wetlands
ELEVATION: 919 feet at trailhead, with no significant rise
ACCESS: Daily, 8 a.m.–10 p.m.; $10 annual recreation passport per vehicle
MAPS: In the information kiosk at the trailhead and at **michigan.gov/dnr**
FACILITIES: Restrooms, picnic area, beach, boat ramp
WHEELCHAIR ACCESS: None
COMMENTS: The trail passes through areas open to seasonal hunting.
CONTACTS: 810-229-6566; **michigan.gov/dnr**

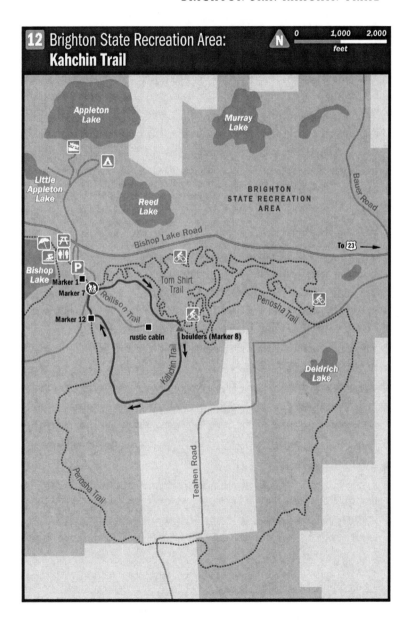

12 Brighton State Recreation Area:
Kahchin Trail

N   0   1,000   2,000
        feet

Appleton
Lake

Murray
Lake

Little
Appleton
Lake

Reed
Lake

BRIGHTON
STATE RECREATION
AREA

Bishop Lake Road

Bauer Road

To 23 →

Bishop
Lake

P

Marker 1

Marker 7

Rollison Trail

Torn Shirt
Trail

Penosha Trail

Marker 12

rustic cabin

boulders (Marker 8)

Kahchin Trail

Deidrich
Lake

Penosha Trail

Teahen Road

Overview

The Kahchin, or Yellow, Trail is the shorter of the two main hiking trails at Brighton State Recreation Area. The trail is a short loop within the longer Penosha, or Blue, Trail (see hike number 13, page 93), covering a similar terrain of rolling woodlands. It's essentially a mini version of the longer trail. In fact, the trail's name, Kahchin, means "short" in the Chippewa language. This is an ideal hike in the fall when the leaves of many of the hardwoods—oaks, maples, and hickory—turn color.

Route Details

Like other state recreation areas in metro Detroit and Ann Arbor, the Brighton State Recreation Area offers a multitude of outdoor activities, including hiking, mountain biking, boating, fishing, swimming, horseback riding, and hunting. The 4,947-acre park also offers rustic cabins and rustic and modern campgrounds for overnight stays. The park is open to hunting in the fall, so hikers are advised to wear bright colors or avoid the trails altogether. Several lakes dot the recreation area, the largest being Bishop Lake in the park's western end. Unfortunately, neither the Kahchin nor the Penosha hiking trails skirt Bishop or any of the other lakes. Both trails, however, do cross through wetlands, a common characteristic of the southeast Michigan landscape.

Both the Kahchin and Penosha trails begin just off the main parking lot for the Bishop Lake day-use area. The trailhead is on the far eastern side of the expansive parking lot. You'll see an information kiosk about 50 feet into the trail on your right. The kiosk displays maps of both trails. For the Kahchin Trail, you'll be following markers 1, 7, 8, and 12. It's an easy-to-follow route, intersecting with the longer Penosha Trail at its beginning and end.

A narrow dirt trail leads into the woods. You'll see a sign denoting a hike-bike trail to your right; it's simply the Penosha Trail, which also is open to mountain bikers. Marker 1 stands at about 112 feet. At this juncture, turn right, heading south to marker 7. Initially, you'll feel as if you're not getting away from the parking area, which remains visible for stretches, but the trail delves deeper into the woods after crossing a park road.

At marker 7, swing left, heading north-northeast to marker 8, about 0.5 miles away. The trail rises slightly and crosses a park road. The woods become thicker as the trail slopes, and you'll notice big oak trees on either side. This is predominantly an oak forest, but you'll also see maple and hickory trees. The Kahchin Trail is simply a walk in the woods; the terrain varies little. En route to marker 8, the trail runs along the crest of a rolling ridge, with a marsh on your left. The trail dips before making its longest climb.

Around this stretch, you'll likely hear an occasional freight train in the distance. Marker 8 stands at the 0.6 -mile mark, where a bench awaits. From here, bear right, heading due south. At this juncture, the trails are no longer shared and the Kahchin Trail should be free of any mountain bikers. The trail is hillier through this stretch and occasionally crosses through small clearings. As you near the 1-mile mark, you'll notice a ravine on your right and cross through wetlands. You'll also see a bench on your right overlooking the ravine.

Marker 12 is near the 1.5-mile mark; the Kahchin and Penosha trails converge at this juncture. Here, swing right, heading north to marker 7 and back to the trailhead. The trail crosses a park road, and the woods thin as you approach the day-use area. A split-rail fence runs along the perimeter of the parking lot as you reach marker 7, at 1.6 miles. Continue straight to the trailhead.

Nearby Attractions

For mountain bikers, Brighton State Recreation Area offers challenging trails, such as the 5.1-mile-long Torn Shirt Mountain Bike Trail, which boasts slow, steep, uphill curves and is heavily wooded. The Murray Lake Trail is 9 miles long; features high, irregular hills; and crosses through grassy marshes. In the summer, downtown

Brighton, about 15 minutes away, hosts outdoor concerts at Mill Pond and farmers' markets on Saturdays. Downtown also boasts a variety of restaurants and shops. The Great Harvest Bread Co. is well known for its variety of homemade breads, cookies, and muffins.

Directions

From Detroit, take I-94 west to M-10, the Lodge Freeway, and take it north. Go about 16 miles to I-696, Exit 18C, toward Lansing. Keep left to follow I-96 to Lansing for 18 miles to Exit 148A, US 23 south to Ann Arbor. Go about 2 miles and take Exit 58, Lee Road. Go west on Lee Road before turning left on Rickett Road. Follow 2 miles and turn right onto Hammel Road. The park entrance is about 0.4 miles on your right.

From Ann Arbor, take US 23 north to Lee Road, Exit 58. Head west on Lee Road and then turn left onto Rickett Road. Go approximately 2 miles and turn right onto Hammel Road. The park entrance is about 0.4 miles on your right.

13 Brighton State Recreation Area:
Penosha Trail

SCENERY: ★ ★ ★
TRAIL CONDITION: ★ ★ ★ ★ ★
CHILDREN: ★ ★
DIFFICULTY: ★ ★ ★
SOLITUDE: ★ ★ ★ ★

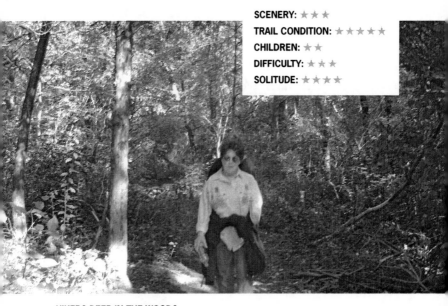

HIKERS DEEP IN THE WOODS

GPS TRAILHEAD COORDINATES: N42° 50.072' W83° 83.466'

DISTANCE & CONFIGURATION: 5-mile loop

HIKING TIME: About 2 hours

HIGHLIGHTS: Rolling woodlands, wetlands

ELEVATION: 919 feet at trailhead, with no significant rise

ACCESS: Daily, 8 a.m.–10 p.m.; $10 annual recreation passport per vehicle

MAPS: At the information kiosk at the trailhead and at **michigan.gov/dnr**

FACILITIES: Restrooms, beach

WHEELCHAIR ACCESS: None

COMMENTS: Portions of the trail cross through areas of the park that are open to seasonal hunting.

CONTACTS: 810-229-6566; **michigan.gov/dnr**

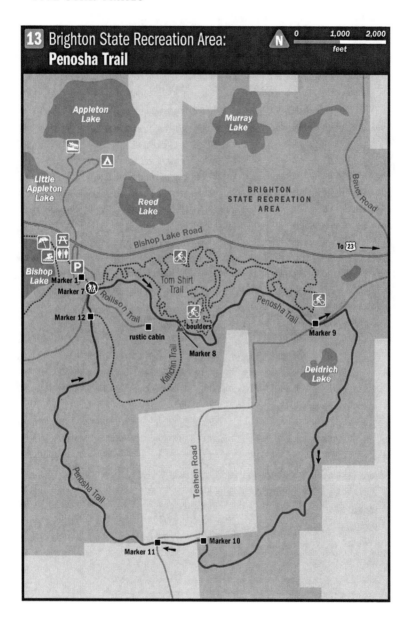

13 Brighton State Recreation Area: **Penosha Trail**

Overview

The longest of the hiking trails at Brighton State Recreation Area in Livingston County, the Penosha Trail (*Penosha* is the Chippewa word for "long") loops through the southeastern section of the 4,947-acre park. The trail passes mostly through hilly woodlands and wetlands (most of the park's lakes are located in other sections), and the sense of wilderness is disrupted only once, deep into the hike, by a short trek along a dirt residential road.

Route Details

Historically, much of the land that comprises the Brighton State Recreation Area was cleared for farming. This landscape of irregular hills, however, proved not conducive to growing crops, and during the Depression, many farmers began selling their unproductive land. The state started purchasing property in earnest for recreation activities in the 1940s.

Today, the park draws hikers, mountain bikers, anglers, beachgoers, equestrians, cross-country skiers, and hunters. Stretches of the trail pass through an area open to hunting in the fall. Hikers are advised to wear bright colors or avoid the trails altogether. Several lakes dot the landscape, but you will pass only one of them, Deidrich Lake, along either the Penosha or the Kahchin trails (see hike 12, page 88), as these paths wind mostly through forests of oak, hickory, and maple.

The trailhead for the Penosha Trail lies just off the far eastern end of the main parking lot at the Bishop Lake day-use area. You'll see an information kiosk about 50 feet into the trail on your right.

Like other state recreation areas, the Penosha Trail uses the state's trail marker system to guide hikers. The trail is well marked, and hikers should follow markers 1, 7, 8, 9, 10, 11, and 12 for this particular hike, or the markers can be followed in the reverse order.

At marker 1, bear right, swinging south and crossing Roilison Trail, a dirt road, before reaching marker 7. The trail slips back into the woods and meanders east and southeast to marker 8, about 0.5 miles from the trailhead. The first of many hills occurs along this stretch but then bottoms out around marker 8. At that junction, continue straight; the trail winds east and northeast from here.

The terrain becomes hillier, and shortly after passing marker 8, you'll notice a remnant from the land's farming past: a long row of boulders used to mark boundaries. Along this stretch, look for a series of wooded hollows created by glaciers. The trail crosses Teahen Road before reaching marker 9. The route from marker 9 to marker 10 presents one of the longest unbroken stretches of the trail—about a mile—passing mostly through rugged woodlands and skirting marshy Deidrich Lake. With the thick foliage, the lake is hard to see most of the year.

Around the 2.5-mile mark, the trail climbs for about 0.3 miles along a thickly wooded ridge to a grassy field. The trail returns to the woods and again climbs to a grassy opening. In late fall, this spot offers panoramic views of the forests. Marker 10 stands around the 3-mile mark. From this junction, the trail runs briefly along Teahen Road. Look for marker 11 about 0.3 miles ahead on the left. A sign notes HIKING TRAIL.

The trail slips back into the woods and then descends toward two ponds. The trail eventually climbs for a long time before reaching an expansive meadow. Marker 12 stands around 4.8 miles. Continue north to marker 7, recrossing Roilison Trail en route to marker 1 and your return to the trailhead.

Nearby Attractions

About 9 miles southeast of the Brighton State Recreation Area is Huron Meadows Metropark, a 1,540-acre expanse that offers limited hiking, fishing, boating, and picnicking. Maltby Lake is the focal point of the park, and a nearly 2-mile hiking trail circles the lake. The southern section of the park straddles the Huron River, with access for canoes and kayakers. However, the trails in this southern section are not well maintained. The park is home to an 18-hole golf course and is a favorite of cross-country skiers in the winter.

Directions

From Detroit, take I-94 west to M-10, the Lodge Freeway, and take it north. Go about 16 miles to I-696, Exit 18C, toward Lansing. Keep left to follow I-96 to Lansing. Follow I-96 for 18 miles to Exit 148A, US 23 south to Ann Arbor. Go about 2 miles and take Exit 58 for Lee Road. Go west on Lee Road before turning left on Rickett Road. Drive 2 miles and turn right onto Hammel Road. The park entrance is about 0.4 miles down, on your right.

From Ann Arbor, take US 23 north to Lee Road, Exit 58. Head west on Lee Road and then turn left onto Rickett Road. Go about 2 miles and turn right onto Hammel Road. The park entrance is about 0.4 miles down, on your right.

14

Island Lake State Recreation Area:
Blue Loop

SCENERY: ★ ★ ★ ★ ★
TRAIL CONDITION: ★ ★ ★ ★
CHILDREN: ★
DIFFICULTY: ★ ★ ★
SOLITUDE: ★ ★ ★

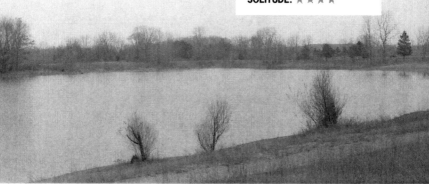

THE EDGE OF THE SPRING MILL CREEK DAY-USE AREA

GPS TRAILHEAD COORDINATES: N42° 30.048' W83° 50.123'

DISTANCE & CONFIGURATION: 9-mile loop

HIKING TIME: About 4 hours

HIGHLIGHTS: Woodlands, Huron River, lakes, wetlands

ELEVATION: 919 feet at trailhead, with no significant rise

ACCESS: Daily, 8 a.m.–10 p.m.; $10 annual recreation passport per vehicle

MAPS: Available from the attendant at the tollbooth or at **michigan.gov/dnr**

FACILITIES: Picnic areas, beach, and restrooms

WHEELCHAIR ACCESS: None

COMMENTS: Portions of the trail cross through areas of the park open to seasonal hunting. Hikers are advised to wear bright colors or to avoid the trail during firearms season in mid- to late November. The trail is extremely busy with bicyclists. Biking is allowed counterclockwise on the trail.

CONTACTS: 810-229-7067; **michigan.gov/dnr**

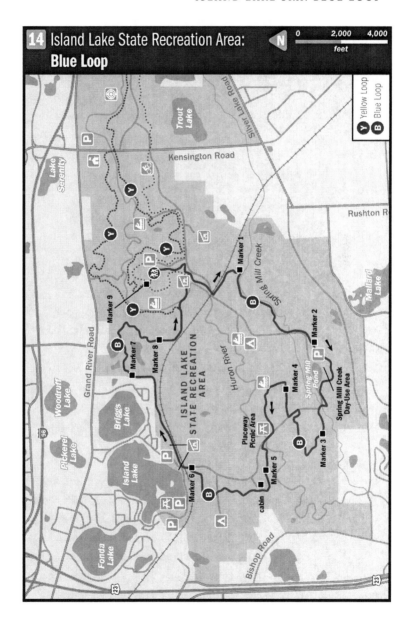

14 Island Lake State Recreation Area:
Blue Loop

N

0   2,000   4,000
feet

Y Yellow Loop
B Blue Loop

Trout Lake

Silver Lake Road

Kensington Road

Lake Serenity

Rushton R

Marker 1

Spring Mill Creek

Mallard Lake

Marker 9

Y

Marker 2

P

Marker 7

B

Grand River Road

Marker 8

ISLAND LAKE STATE RECREATION AREA

Huron River

Marker 4

Spring Mill Pond

Spring Mill Creek Day-Use Area

Woodruff Lake

Briggs Lake

Placeway Picnic Area

Marker 3

B

96

Pickerel Lake

Island Lake

Marker 5

Marker 6

B

cabin

Fonda Lake

P

23

Bishop Road

23

Overview

The longest of the hiking trails at Island Lake State Recreation Area, the Blue Loop traverses deeper into the park but covers much of the same terrain as the shorter Yellow Loop (see hike 15, page 103). The landscape is a blend of rugged woodlands, wetlands, and creeks. The Blue Loop also passes through day-use areas near Island Lake and Spring Mill Creek.

Route Details

Formerly known as the West Loop, the Blue Loop shares the same trailhead with the shorter Yellow Loop. The trailhead is located at the northwest corner of the parking lot off Park Road.

Both trails are clearly marked by yellow and blue dots atop signposts. As both are open to multiuse, expect to share the trails with mountain bikers and trail runners. The trails converge only for a short stretch along a narrow dirt path that immediately leads into the woods, thick with brush on either side.

The sense of Michigan's Up North is accentuated by sandy stretches, thick woods, and stands of white pines and other evergreens. After about 500 feet, the trails diverge after crossing a paved park road and a bench. The Yellow Loop veers to the right. The Blue Loop continues to the left, heading south.

Although the Blue Loop is much longer than the Yellow Loop, the terrain varies little. For the most part, the trail travels under the canopy of hardwood forests and along rugged terrain. Occasional meadows dot the trail, and the sense of solitude is disrupted only at the day-use area at Spring Mill Creek, at Island Lake, and along a cargo rail line. The Spring Mill Creek day-use area is busy in the summer months with beachgoers; Island Lake is a popular picnic spot in the spring, summer, and fall; and freight trains pass through the park three or four times a day.

Once the Blue Loop separates from the Yellow Loop, the trail runs parallel to a park road. After crossing park roads twice, the trail slips back into the woods and rises above the Huron River, the waterway barely visible through the trees. Around the 0.5-mile mark, the trail again crosses a park road, as well as railroad tracks. An aluminum fence runs along the track on your left. The trail then runs southeast into the woods and across wetlands.

Over the next mile, the trail turns southwest and runs along Spring Mill Creek and then parallels the park road as it meanders toward the Spring Mill Creek day-use area. Then expect a long open stretch, with the park road on your right. The trail becomes more gravel than dirt, and the parking lot and day-use area will be visible on your right as well.

After passing the Spring Mill Creek day-use area, the trail crosses the creek and winds back in the woods, heading west and then northeast to the Placeway Picnic Area. Notice the deep ravines along this stretch. The trail crosses the park road again around the 3.5-mile mark and reaches the Placeway Picnic Area 0.5 miles later.

The trail again borders the park road before crossing the Huron River and then swings westward. This section offers another heavily wooded, hilly stretch, with deep ravines, occasional fields and meadows, and scattered pines. As the trail approaches the Island Lake day-use area, it swings east and follows a railroad line. The trail continues easterly, bypassing the day-use area and remaining on the north side of the Huron River, following the rail line for about 0.5 miles.

Around 6.5 miles, the trail swings to the left, heading north and descending into a field and past houses. The trail is back in the woods within 0.8 miles and crosses the Huron River near 8.3 miles. The trail swings westward, heading back to the trailhead.

Nearby Attractions

If you're up for a less-strenuous walk, the Huron Valley Rail Trail (about 5 miles southeast of the park) makes for a pleasant trek from South Lyon to Milford Road. The 3.5-mile portion of the point-to-point trail, formerly an old rail line, is accessible off 10 Mile Road, on the eastern edge of South Lyon and adjacent to the railroad tracks that run through the town. The trail is mostly lined with trees, crosses through light woods, and passes by South Lyon High School, some subdivisions, and horse farms. South Lyon's downtown is within walking distance from the 10 Mile Road parking lot and is home to boutique shops, restaurants, coffee shops, and a movie theater.

Directions

From Detroit, take I-75 north to westbound I-696. I-696 turns into I-96 at the I-275 interchange (stay in the left lane). Continue on I-96 west for about 15 miles; take Exit 151 for Kensington Road. Head south on Kensington Road and follow it about 0.3 miles past the light at Grand River Avenue. The park entrance is on the left. Turn right after the entrance booth and follow the road to the second right (Park Road) after the two stop signs at the bridge. The road leads to the trailhead parking lot.

From Ann Arbor, take US 23 north from M-14 about 15 miles to I-96 eastbound. Follow I-96 about 3.5 miles to Kensington Road, Exit 151. Turn right and drive to the park entrance on the left-hand side. Turn right after the entrance booth and follow the road to the second right (Park Road) after the two stop signs at the bridge. The road leads to the trailhead parking lot.

15

Island Lake State Recreation Area:
Yellow Loop

SCENERY: ★ ★ ★
TRAIL CONDITION: ★ ★ ★ ★
CHILDREN: ★ ★
DIFFICULTY: ★ ★ ★
SOLITUDE: ★ ★ ★

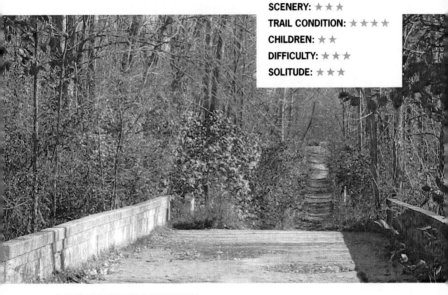

A BRIDGE CROSSES A WATERWAY.

GPS TRAILHEAD COORDINATES: N42° 50.820' W83° 70.842'

DISTANCE & CONFIGURATION: 6-mile loop

HIKING TIME: About 3 hours

HIGHLIGHTS: Woodlands, rolling hills, fields, Huron River

ELEVATION: 928 feet at trailhead, with no significant rise

ACCESS: Daily, 8 a.m.–10 p.m.; $10 annual recreation passport per vehicle

MAPS: Available from the attendant at the tollbooth and at **michigan.gov/dnr**

FACILITIES: Restrooms, picnic area

WHEELCHAIR ACCESS: None

COMMENTS: The Island Lake State Recreation Area trails are extremely crowded with mountain bikers on weekends. They are allowed to ride counterclockwise on the trail. To avoid a constant parade of bikers, it's best to hike the trail on weekdays.

CONTACTS: 810-229-7067; **michigan.gov/dnr**

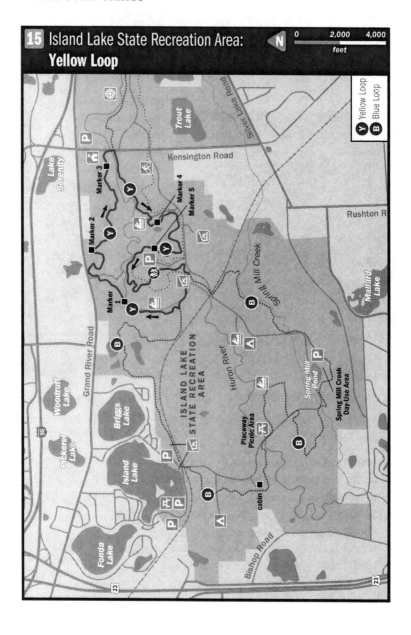

15 Island Lake State Recreation Area:
Yellow Loop

Overview

Formerly known as the East Loop, the renamed Yellow Loop circles a winding stretch of the Huron River, passing through mature woods, meadows, fields, and wetlands. Occasionally, the trail follows and rises above the river line, offering lovely views of the waterway. The trail is well marked and easy to follow, with distance markers posted along the way. There can be long stretches of solitude, but don't be surprised by the frequent interaction with mountain bikers.

Route Details

Despite its proximity to I-96, just 0.5 miles away, Island Lake State Recreation Area captures the sense of wilderness of northern Michigan. The 4,000-acre park is home to mature hardwood forests, meadows, winding rivers and creeks, lakes, and gently rolling hills. Plenty of recreational opportunities exist for outdoor enthusiasts, including biking, canoeing, boating, fishing, and hunting. The recreation area also is home to a shooting range (in a self-contained area in another section of the park), so don't be surprised to hear the sounds of guns while you're traipsing through the woods.

The Yellow Loop is the shorter of the park's two main hiking trails (the other is the Blue Loop; see hike 14, page 98). It meanders all around the scenic Huron River and crosses the waterway in two spots. The feeling of backcountry is broken only on occasion whenever the trail crosses park roads and parallels Old Grand River Avenue. For the most part, the Yellow Loop runs deep in the woods and under the canopy of hardwood trees.

The trailhead stands at the northwest corner of the parking lot off Park Road. Both the Yellow and Blue loops begin at the trailhead. Both trails are clearly marked, with yellow and blue dots atop signposts. Both are open to multiuse, so expect to share the trails with mountain bikers and trail runners. A narrow dirt trail leads immediately into the woods and past stands of white pines and evergreens. The Yellow and Blue trails diverge after about 500 feet, after crossing a paved park road and passing a bench.

The Yellow Loop then swings to the left, and bends and slopes downward, away from the paved road. It passes through another stand of pines before coming to a small clearing at about 0.4 miles. You will see a parking lot on the left. As the dirt trail widens, bike and deer and other animal tracks become more noticeable, a reminder that you're likely to share stretches of the trail. The trail passes a marsh before reaching a cement bridge that crosses the Huron River, slow-moving in the late summer and fall.

Bear right at the next intersection. The trail widens and becomes sandy as it follows the riverbank, occasionally affording scenic views as the trees thin. The trail eventually narrows and rises with the terrain, and the woods become thick with yellow maples. As the trail descends, the river and floodplain become more visible.

The trail follows the riverbank for a long stretch. A cluster of white pines stands near the 1.3-mile mark, where a long wooden bridge crosses Mann Creek, and the trail lines the opposite bank for another 0.3 miles. Long before Kensington Road comes into view, you'll hear the buzz of cars and trucks. You'll eventually catch a glimpse of I-96 as well. As the trail climbs above the road, Kent Lake becomes visible in the distance. The trail now veers southwestward, passing through more woods and occasional clearings with clusters of white pines, small trees, and cedars.

At the 3-mile mark, the wide gravel trail veers right and parallels the road before crossing a long wooden bridge over the Huron River, the second and final crossing. The trail climbs above the river for about 0.3 miles before opening to sprawling fields broken only by an occasional majestic tree. You will spot the roofs of farm outbuildings on the horizon. The trail runs between fields and lines of trees for about 0.5 miles. Around the 3.8-mile marker, look for a stop sign and dirt road crossing. Over the next mile, the trail runs along expansive stretches of swamps and marshes. The trail eventually veers away from the marshy areas and back into hilly wooded terrain. At the

5.5-mile marker, the trail crosses a bike path. From here, hikers will retrace their steps, as the Yellow and Blue loop trails converge, and return to the trailhead.

Nearby Attractions

On the other side of I-96 lies Kensington Metropark. The park boasts more than 1,200 acres of water surrounded by rolling, wooded hills. A paved trail rims the perimeter of the lake and attracts bikers and inline skaters. While the park is busy with walkers, bikers, inline skaters, and water enthusiasts, a nature study area offers a respite from the crowds with seven hiking trails that traverse wetlands, forests, and fields. The most rustic are the 1-mile-long Chickadee Loop and the 0.5-mile-long Fox Trail (see hike 16, page 108).

Directions

From Detroit, take I-75 north to westbound I-696. I-696 turns into I-96 at the I-275 interchange (stay in the left lane). Continue on I-96 west for about 15 miles to Kensington Road, Exit 151. Head south on Kensington Road and follow it about 0.3 miles past the light at Grand River Avenue. The park entrance is on the left. Turn right after the entrance booth and follow the road to the second right (Park Road) after the two stop signs at the bridge. The road leads to the trailhead parking lot.

From Ann Arbor, take US 23 north from M-14 about 15 miles to I-96 eastbound. Follow it about 3.5 miles to Kensington Road, Exit 151. Turn right and drive to the park entrance on the left-hand side. Turn right after the entrance booth and follow the road to the second right (Park Road) after the two stop signs at the bridge. The road leads to the trailhead parking lot.

16

Kensington Metropark:
Deer Run, Fox, and Chickadee Trails

SCENERY: ★ ★ ★
TRAIL CONDITION: ★ ★ ★ ★ ★
CHILDREN: ★ ★ ★
DIFFICULTY: ★ ★
SOLITUDE: ★ ★ ★

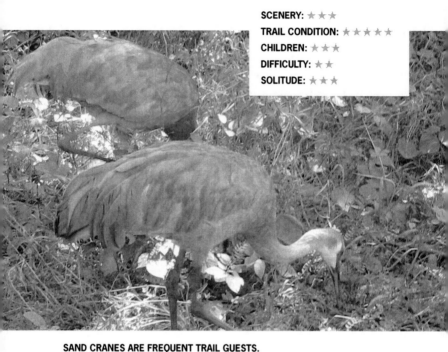

SAND CRANES ARE FREQUENT TRAIL GUESTS.

GPS TRAILHEAD COORDINATES: N42° 31.710' W83° 40.180'

DISTANCE & CONFIGURATION: 1.8-mile loop

HIKING TIME: About 1 hour or less

HIGHLIGHTS: Woods, fields, remnants of an ancient bog

ELEVATION: 870 feet at trailhead, with no significant rise

ACCESS: Daily, 6 a.m.–10 p.m. Nature center: Monday, 1–5 p.m.; Tuesday–Sunday, 10 a.m.–5 p.m.; $5 per day or $25 per year

MAPS: At the nature center and **metroparks.com**

FACILITIES: Nature center, restrooms, picnic area

WHEELCHAIR ACCESS: Deer Run Trail—yes; Fox and Chickadee trails—no

COMMENTS: This is the busiest park in the metropark system and the state, and the nature trails are well used.

CONTACTS: 248-685-0603; **metroparks.com**

Overview

The Deer Run Trail loops through woods and marshlands in the northeastern section of the 700-acre nature center property. A boardwalk cuts through an ancient bog and offers a shortcut for hikers who don't want to do the entire length. The distance covered here includes adding the Fox Trail and an arm of the Chickadee Loop, which are two of the nature center's more remote and less-traveled trails. Their addition provides for a deeper trek into thick woods.

Route Details

The second-oldest park in the metropark system, Kensington is home to acres of wooded hills, expansive meadows, tamarack swamps, bogs, Kent Lake, and the winding Huron River. Kent Lake, originally 60 acres, expanded to 1,200 acres due to land-clearing and river damming. Boaters and anglers enjoy the lake, and its beaches, Martindale and Maple, lure thousands of beachgoers in the summer.

You can see Kent Lake from the beginning of Deer Run Trail, which runs by Kingfisher Lagoon, outside the nature center. But none of the nature trails come close to the lake.

The Deer Run Trail, which ranges in length from 1.3 to 1.8 miles, depending on whether you use the trail's shortcut, is one of three trails at the nature center that stretch deep into the woods, which are mostly second-growth forests of beech and maple. Some old-growth oaks can be spotted here and there. Much of the land was cleared for farming and development, though sprawling oaks were left for fence lines and shade. The 0.5-mile Fox Trail and the 1-mile Chickadee Loop are accessible from the northern loop of Deer Run. Adding these trails makes for an enjoyable, longer trek of 1.8 miles, and both pretty much run under the cover of the woods.

Like the other trails, Deer Run begins right outside the rear entrance of the nature center. Turn right, heading northeast. In the warm months, notice the odd marker at the beginning—a purple spaceshiplike structure. It's a contraption for emerald ash borers,

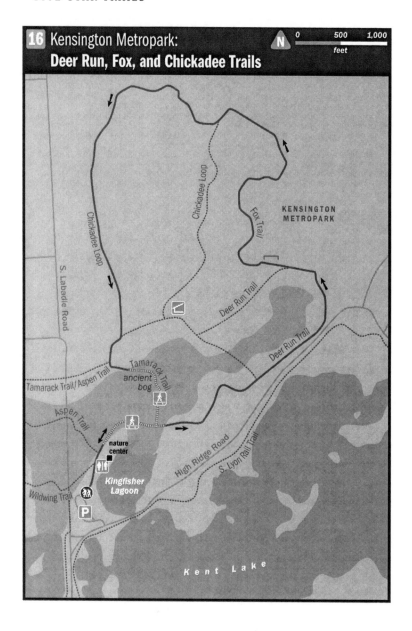

16 Kensington Metropark:
Deer Run, Fox, and Chickadee Trails

N

0   500   1,000
feet

KENSINGTON
METROPARK

Chickadee Loop

Chickadee Loop

Fox Trail

Deer Run Trail

Deer Run Trail

S. Labadie Road

Tamarack Trail

Tamarack Trail/Aspen Trail

ancient
bog

Aspen Trail

nature
center

High Ridge Road

S. Lyon Rail Trail

Kingfisher
Lagoon

Wildwing Trail

P

Kent Lake

which were responsible for the destruction of more than 25 million ash trees in Michigan and other states, and it's part of a study by the U.S. Department of Agriculture.

The dirt and gravel path immediately cuts through marshlands and over a series of small boardwalks as it heads northeast. Kent Lake becomes visible through the trees. Expect to see and hear cars, as this part of the trail runs parallel to a park road.

Eventually, the trail winds away from the park road, turning northwest. Early-morning hikers stand a good chance of observing birds, including nighthawks, fly catchers, swallows, snipes, and woodcocks. Wildlife is plentiful too. White-tailed deer and wild turkeys are common. Hikers often find the tracks of mink, coyotes, and foxes on the trail.

The first intersection offers hikers a shortcut through an ancient bog. Avoid the shortcut and continue straight, heading northeast. The landscape remains the same, and the second intersection, the **Fox Trail,** comes just after you cross a small bridge over a creek. The creek flows year-round and often compels hikers to linger here on a bench to enjoy the beauty and tranquility. Swing right on the Fox Trail, heading northeast and northwest as the trail zigzags through woods and meadows. Watch for piles of rocks that once served as fence lines when the land was farmed. Just before you pass a small pond on your left at the top of a hill, be aware that a path running off the trail is for access to a gas pipe; a sign marks that intention, but many hikers often become confused here and inadvertently follow that path. If that happens to you, just turn around and retrace your steps away from the gas pipe.

The Fox Trail ends at a T-intersection at Chickadee Loop. Turn left, heading south back to the Deer Run Trail. This sometimes hilly stretch along the Chickadee Loop is among the most beautiful in the park, running deep into a second-growth forest. In autumn, this section is brilliant with the colors of aspen, sumac, and sassafras trees.

To complete your three-trail loop, you will return to Deer Run Trail, rejoining the trail near a shelter on your left. Turn right on Deer Run, which merges with the Tamarack Trail, as its heads west back to the nature center. Signs will help show the way.

Nearby Attractions

The picturesque village of Milford lies on Milford Road, off the eastern entrance of Kensington Metropark. Its Main Street exudes small-town charm and is lined with restaurants, cafés, and boutiques. The village also boasts six parks, and within walking distance of the business district, its Central Park sits on the banks of the Huron River. The park features a playground and basketball and tennis courts, and outfitters offer kayak rentals in the warm months. The park also has a picnic area and is home to summer concerts.

Directions

From Detroit, take I-75 north to I-696 west, Exit 61. After about 18 miles, I-696 merges into I-96 west toward Lansing. Continue another 8 miles, to Exit 155B. Go 2.7 miles and turn left onto Huron River Parkway, the park entrance. Follow the signs to the nature center.

From Ann Arbor, take US 23 north to I-96, Exit 60A, toward Detroit. Exit at Kensington Road, Exit 151. Turn right on Kensington Road, and then right onto Highridge Drive, the western entrance to the park. Follow the signs to the nature center.

17

Kensington Metropark:
Wildwing Trail

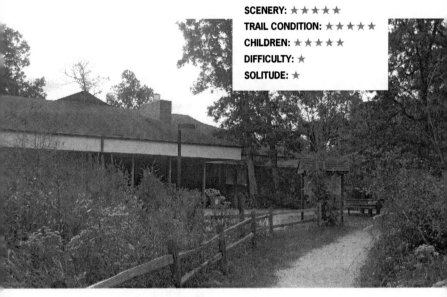

SCENERY: ★ ★ ★ ★ ★
TRAIL CONDITION: ★ ★ ★ ★ ★
CHILDREN: ★ ★ ★ ★ ★
DIFFICULTY: ★
SOLITUDE: ★

THE TRAILHEAD AT THE NATURE CENTER

GPS TRAILHEAD COORDINATES: N42° 31.710' W83° 40.180'

DISTANCE & CONFIGURATION: 2-mile loop

HIKING TIME: About 1 hour or less

HIGHLIGHTS: Woods, Wildwing Lake, osprey hacking tower

ELEVATION: 870 feet at trailhead, with no significant rise

ACCESS: Daily, 6 a.m.–10 p.m. Nature center: Monday, 1–5 p.m.; Tuesday–Sunday, 10 a.m.–5 p.m.; $5 per day or $25 per year

MAPS: At the nature center and **metroparks.com**

FACILITIES: Nature center, restrooms, picnic area

WHEELCHAIR ACCESS: Yes

COMMENTS: This is not only the busiest park in the metropark system but also in the state, attracting more than 1 million visitors a year. Because of Wildwing Lake, the board-walk, and its proximity to the nature center, the Wildwing Trail is one of the more popular hiking trails in the park; don't expect to find solitude.

CONTACTS: 248-685-0603; **metroparks.com**

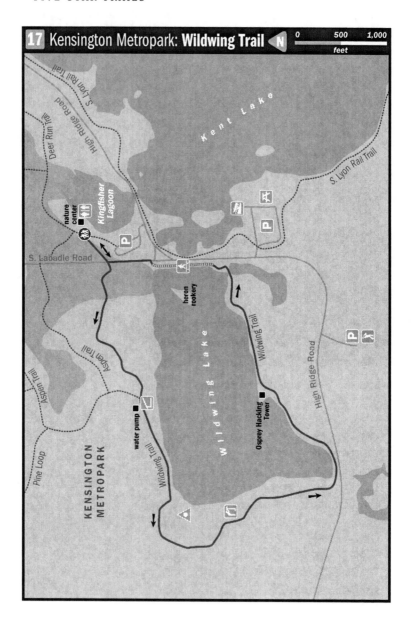

17 Kensington Metropark: **Wildwing Trail**

Overview

The nature center's longest trail, the Wildwing Trail, is easy to follow as it loops around Wildwing Lake. Ample opportunities exist to see aquatic life, such as muskrats and snapping turtles, as well as waterfowl, including geese and swans. Many visitors come to catch glimpses of migrant songbirds, as well as ospreys and herons. Don't be surprised to find photographers around the osprey hacking tower on any given day.

Route Details

It's easy to see why the Wildwing Trail is the most popular of the seven trails at the Kensington Metropark Nature Center. It's an easy-to-follow and gentle trail that crosses wetlands and meadows as it wraps around Wildwing Lake. The expansive views of the lake—not to mention aquatic life and birds—draw lots of families.

Like the other trails at the nature center, the Wildwing Trail begins just outside the rear entrance. Swing left and head southwest, past the first intersection with the Aspen Trail. The trail become becomes a wide dirt swath, and it's not uncommon along this stretch to encounter sand cranes, which draw the curious.

Within 1,000 feet, the trail comes to a four-way intersection. Continue straight, heading west and past a rock display on your right. The trail crosses through marshes, thick with cattails and reeds on either side. Wildflowers abound along this stretch, and you'll notice tamaracks dotting the marshlands.

At the next junction, you'll find a water pump—no longer functioning but once offering drinking water—and a shelter. The trail on your right, heading north, is another arm of the Aspen Trail. Continue straight, heading west-southwest. A bench invites a moment to sit and observe the lake.

You'll encounter no other intersecting trails until you've traversed the length of Wildwing Lake and crossed a long boardwalk at its eastern end.

From the bench, the Wildwing Trail passes through meadows, slight woodlands, and marshes as it winds around the lake. Tunneling prairie moles are common in the meadows; expect to see lots of field sparrows. The lake is often visible through the trees, and at about the halfway point, a deck with benches overlooks the entire lake. The lake is double its original size. During the creation of the metropark, officials expanded the lake eastward when they dammed the Huron River to create adjacent Kent Lake. Because the western half of the lake predates the park, ice fishing is allowed. Anglers come to hook northern pike and perch.

Heading south from the overlook is a steep hill. Another trail highlight includes traversing along a gravel hill, deposited by glaciers thousands of years ago; the gravel helps filter water flowing into the lake. The osprey hacking tower on the southern shoreline was part of the state's efforts to reintroduce the fish-eating birds back to southeastern Michigan. In the late 1990s, the park became home to the first nesting pair of ospreys in the region since the 1960s. A long boardwalk crosses through marshland on the lake's eastern edge before the trail returns to the nature center.

Nearby Attractions

One of the oldest parks in the metropark system, Kensington offers something for everyone all year long. The 4,481-acre park's amenities include hiking, biking, picnicking, horseback riding, swimming, boating, and golfing. In the winter, visitors come here to ice skate, sled, cross-country ski, and ice fish. The park is a frequent destination for family outings, not only because of the beach and swimming opportunities but also for the Farm Learning Center and the nature center. The 100-acre Farm Learning Center borders the Huron River. The reconstructed barn and grounds are home to a variety of domestic animals, including cows, pigs, sheep, goats, chickens, and rabbits. The grounds include herb and crop gardens, and interpreters are on hand to explain farm life. At the nature center, the Pine Loop is the newest trail and begins off the Aspen Trail; its notable feature is a vernal pond visible in the spring. It's also a great spot to catch roosting great horned owls.

An 8-mile paved trail loops around Kent Lake, passing along picnic and playground areas. The trail connects to the Huron Valley Rail Trail, which heads south to South Lyon, ending at 10 Mile Road, and north to Wixom. In South Lyon, about 5 miles southeast, Erwin Orchards and Cider Mill on Pontiac Trail is a popular fall destination. The mill sells freshly made apple cider, homemade doughnuts, and apples. The grounds include a playground. Raspberry picking is available in late summer.

Directions

From Detroit, take I-75 north to I-696 west, Exit 61. After about 18 miles, I-696 merges into I-96 west toward Lansing. Continue another 8 miles; exit at 155B. Go 2.7 miles and turn left onto Huron River Parkway, the entrance to the park. Follow the signs to the nature center.

From Ann Arbor, take US 23 north to I-96, Exit 60A, toward Detroit. Take Exit 151, Kensington Road. Turn right on Kensington Road, and then right onto Highridge Drive, the western entrance to the park. Follow the signs to the nature center.

18 # Lakelands Trail
State Park

SCENERY: ★ ★
TRAIL CONDITION: ★ ★ ★ ★ ★
CHILDREN: ★ ★ ★
DIFFICULTY: ★
SOLITUDE: ★ ★ ★ ★

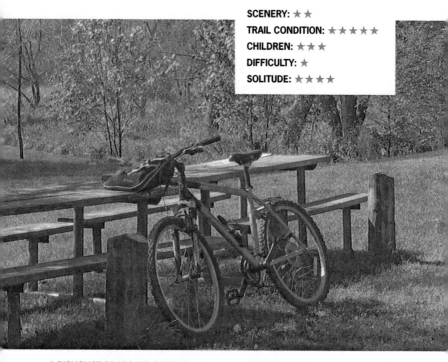

A BICYCLIST PROPS HIS GEAR AT A PICNIC TABLE NEAR GREGORY.

GPS TRAILHEAD COORDINATES: N42° 27.652' W83° 56.519'

DISTANCE & CONFIGURATION: 7.6 mile point-to-point with shuttle

HIKING TIME: About 3 hours

HIGHLIGHTS: Woods, wetlands, rolling farmland

ELEVATION: 915 feet at trailhead, with no significant rise

ACCESS: Open 24/7; no fees or permits required

MAPS: At the trailhead and **michigan.gov/dnr**

FACILITIES: None

WHEELCHAIR ACCESS: Yes

COMMENTS: Horses and bicycles are allowed on some stretches of the trail. For shuttle purposes for the hike described here, you can park at the Pinckney and Gregory trailheads.

CONTACTS: 734-426-4913; **michigan.gov/dnr**

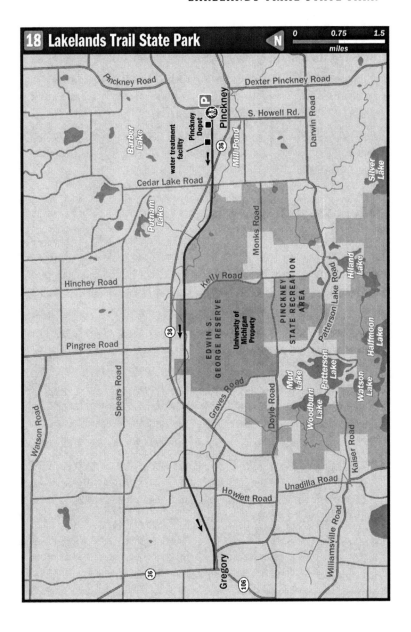

18 Lakelands Trail State Park

Overview

Running east and west along an abandoned railroad line, this portion of the Lakelands Trail State Park passes through rolling farmland, woodlands, and wetlands. The gentle trail frequently crosses rural roads and small creeks and runs parallel to M-36. Thin woods line most of the trail, but there are patches of open fields and occasional houses. The communities of Pinckney and Gregory bookend this section of the trail.

Route Details

One of four linear parks in Michigan's state park system, Lakelands stretches 13 miles from Pinckney to Stockbridge; this trek focuses on about half the trail, from Pinckney to Gregory. The multiuse trail is familiar to hikers, bikers, equestrians, and cross-country skiers. Hiking and biking are encouraged on the north side of the trail; horseback riding is welcomed on the south along some stretches, where equestrian paths intersect the main trail.

The trailhead in Pinckney is off a dirt parking lot on the west side of D-19, about 0.5 miles north of M-36. An apartment building stands on the opposite side of the street, and the abandoned Pinckney Depot is located on the north side of the trail.

As you head west, the trail immediately passes industrial buildings on the left, and there's a thin line of trees on either side. From Pinckney to Gregory, at about the halfway mark of the entire 13-mile trail, the landscape varies with woodlands, open fields and meadows, rolling farmland, and the occasional home and farm buildings.

Around the 0.3-mile mark, the trail crosses a paved dead-end street. The town's water treatment facilities are on the right, and after crossing the street, you'll find another small building on your right—also part of the water treatment facility. From here, the woods on either side become thicker and you'll pass fewer homes and buildings. The trail crosses a field lined with power lines around the 1-mile mark and then a horse farm and a cluster of houses before crossing M-36.

Within 0.3 miles, the trail crosses a dirt road—a house is on the left—and slips back into woodlands. Wetlands border either side, and around the 1.5-mile mark, a small wooden bridge crosses a creek. The first of a series of intersections with horse trails can be seen on your left near the 1.8-mile mark. A bench is on your right. Another small bridge crosses a creek near the 2-mile mark.

Over the next mile, the trail crosses over a couple of small bridges and passes through wetlands and power lines on your right. You'll see a farm on your left as you reach the 3-mile mark. About 0.2 miles later, the trail crosses a dirt road and then passes along a long line of white pine trees on your right, shielding a house. A large oak tree stands on the south side of the trail next to a fence protecting the Edwin S. George Reserve, a 1,500-acre University of Michigan biological research area.

Signs mark a private driveway that crosses the trail just before you reach 4 miles. Both sides of the trail become thick with brush and low-lying shrubs. The scenery changes little along this stretch. You'll reach M-36 again at the 4.8-mile mark.

At 0.3 miles later, a dirt road intersects the trail. The trail then passes under a canopy of tall beeches, maples, and oaks before returning to open fields and wetlands. From here to Gregory, the trail passes a driveway and intersects with a pair of dirt roads and an occasional farm. The trail reaches Gregory around the 7.4-mile mark. You'll walk behind a gas station and pizza eatery on your left and a bank on your right as you reach M-36, the end of the one-way 7.6-mile hike. Gregory is a good ending point, with parking, stores, and restaurants nearby. While there is no designated parking area to leave your car as a shuttle in Gregory, ample parking is available in the lots of surrounding businesses. To get to Gregory, travel west along M-36 from Pinckney. M-36 swings north as it runs through Gregory. To continue to Stockton, the western end of the 13-mile trail, cross M-36 and continue west.

Nearby Attractions

It's hard not to be intrigued by the community of Hell, about 3.5 miles southwest of Lakelands Trail State Park. Just a cluster of buildings along M-36, Hell has gained notoriety thanks to the Travel Channel and a variety of national advertising campaigns. With a population of about 225, the community is home to a general store, miniature golf course, bar, and gas station. Events throughout the year take advantage of the town's frightening name.

Directions

From Detroit, take I-75 north to I-696 west (Exit 61) toward Lansing. Merge onto I-96 west toward Lansing. Follow it about 16 miles to US 23 south, Exit 148. Go about 4 miles to Exit 55 for Silver Lake Road. Turn right on Silver Lake Road, go 0.1 mile, and then turn left on Whitmore Lake Road. Go about 0.2 miles and turn right onto Winans Lake Road and drive 2 miles. Turn left on Hamburg Road and go 0.5 miles. Turn right on M-36 and drive about 8 miles to Pinckney. Turn right on D-19. The parking lot to the trail is about 0.5 miles north on your left.

From Ann Arbor, take US 23 north to Exit 54B, toward Pinckney. Turn a slight right onto M-36/Nine Mile Road and follow it west to Pinckney, about 11 miles. Turn right onto D-19. The parking lot for the trail is about 0.5 mile north on your left.

See Route Details for directions to Gregory, where you can leave your car as a shuttle.

Proud Lake State Recreation Area:
River Trail

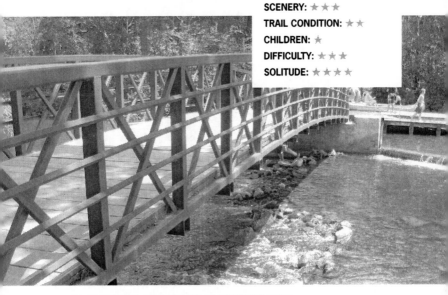

SCENERY: ★ ★ ★
TRAIL CONDITION: ★ ★
CHILDREN: ★
DIFFICULTY: ★ ★ ★
SOLITUDE: ★ ★ ★ ★

A BRIDGE CROSSES OVER A POPULAR SWIMMING HOLE.

GPS TRAILHEAD COORDINATES: N42° 34.437' W83° 33.516'

DISTANCE & CONFIGURATION: 5.7-mile loop

HIKING TIME: About 3 hours

HIGHLIGHTS: Woodlands, Huron River, red pine plantation

ELEVATION: 903 feet at trailhead, with no significant rise

ACCESS: Daily, 8 a.m.–10 p.m.; $10 annual recreation passport per vehicle

MAPS: Available from the attendant at the tollbooth and park headquarters off Wixom Road, and **michigan.gov/dnr**

FACILITIES: Camping, picnic tables, restrooms, boat ramp

WHEELCHAIR ACCESS: None

COMMENTS: Portions of the trail cross through areas of the park open to seasonal hunting. Be advised to wear orange vests or avoid the trail altogether during firearms season for deer in mid- to late November.

CONTACTS: 248-685-2433; **michigan.gov/dnr**

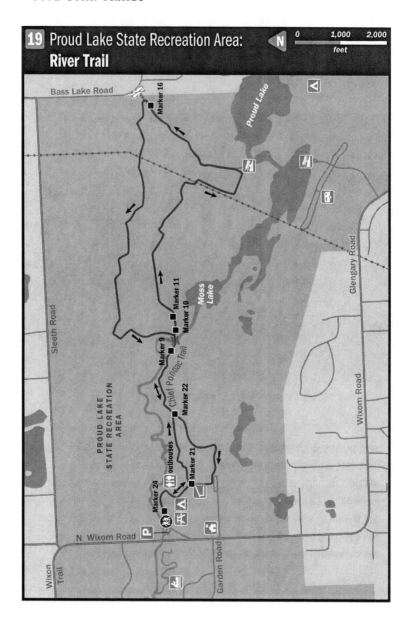

19 Proud Lake State Recreation Area:
River Trail

Overview

The River Trail crosses through a huge swath of the Proud Lake State Recreation Area, giving hikers a good sense of the park's varied landscape. The trail initially runs along the wooded southern banks of the Huron River and then moves into rolling woodlands and marshlands. The trail also crosses an unusual dam that forms Moss Lake, an area that lures lots of kayakers, swimmers, and anglers. As the trail nears its end, it passes through a red pine plantation.

Route Details

With its rolling dense woodlands, expansive wetlands, and a chain of small lakes, Proud Lake State Recreation Area attracts a variety of outdoor enthusiasts. The Huron River also winds through the 4,700-acre park in southwestern Oakland County. The park is named after the biggest of the lakes, Proud Lake. The lake is visible from this trail as it loops at the far eastern end.

The trailhead to the River Trail is located at a fishing access site just north of the park headquarters off Wixom Road. A small dirt parking lot fronts the Huron River, and during the busy summer months, an attendant staffs the entrance. The trail begins in the northeast corner of the parking lot and immediately slips eastward into the woods and runs parallel to the Huron River for about 0.3 miles. The trail then swings inland and crosses a clearing with a pair of outhouses, part of a group campground area. A spur leads to a campground. The trail is not well marked in this section, but just continue past the outhouses, and then swing left (east).

Around the 0.5-mile mark, you'll cross a path on your right that leads to the day-use area and the Marsh Trail. Continue heading straight (east). You will see the signposts used by Michigan's state trail marker system when you come to marker 21 near the 0.8-mile mark. At this junction, bear left, continuing east. In late May, this stretch is known for blooming marsh marigolds. Yellow birches also are scattered in the surrounding woods, and this is a good spot to encounter wildlife, such as white-tailed deer.

This stretch is also known as the Chief Pontiac Trail, and you'll find interpretive signs along the route identifying tree and plant species and explaining how Native Americans used them. The trail cuts through extensive wetlands, and it can be very muddy in the spring and fall.

Around the 1-mile mark, the trail passes through an open camping area with access to the river. Just ahead is the Huron River Dam. Cross the bridge and bear right—marker 10 is there on the opposite side of the river. Marker 11 is about 0.2 miles ahead.

Most of the trail on this side of the river is thick with woods and is more rugged. The trail heads northeast on its way to its eastern end and spills out onto a dirt road for a short distance. Look for marker 12, around the 1.4-mile mark.

Around the 2-mile mark, the trail splits. Continue straight, heading east-southeast. Within about 0.3 miles, the trail passes through a field and row of power lines and then dips back into the woods. Look for marker 15 around the 2.4-mile mark; in less than another 0.3 miles, you'll arrive at a dirt access road to Proud Lake. You'll see the lake and boat ramp on your right. Turn left and follow the dirt-gravel road north-northeast for about 0.5 miles.

Just before reaching a yellow road access gate, you'll see the trail on your left and marker 16. You'll also see a NO DUMPING sign on your left. A small bridge crosses a creek, and the trail follows a low ridgeline before running under the power lines again. Back in the woods, the trail continues north-northwest, intersecting with another trail around the 3.5-mile mark. Continue straight. It's a long stretch with the rugged woodlands before returning to the dam 1 mile later.

From the dam, retrace your steps along the Chief Pontiac Trail but swing left (south) at marker 22 to marker 20. The trail passes between towering red pine trees, planted decades ago as part of a plantation. At the trailhead, walk through the parking lot to the campground and then cut west to return to the River Trail. Swing left and follow the trail back to the trailhead.

Nearby Attractions

About 6 miles southeast of the recreation area and south of I-96 is Lyon Oaks County Park, one of several parks in the Oakland County system. The 1,043-acre park features a golf course, bark park, nature center, and an interesting network of trails, some still being developed. The park's current 3.6 miles of trails meander through woods and wetlands, home to coyotes, red and gray foxes, mink, white-tailed deer, and Michigan's only venomous snake, the massasauga rattler. The park also is a magnet for bird-watchers, who come to observe spring migrations, particularly of warblers.

Directions

From Detroit, take I-75 north to Exit 61 for I-696 west toward Lansing. I-696 merges into I-96. Continue west to Exit 159, Wixom Road North. Go about 0.5 miles and merge onto South Wixom Road. Drive about 4 miles and turn left onto North Wixom Road. Go about 1.7 miles to the access site on your right.

From Ann Arbor, take US 23 north to Exit 60A, I-96 east toward Detroit. Follow that to Exit 159, Wixom Road. Bear left onto Wixom Road North. Go about 4 miles and turn left onto North Wixom Road. Go about 1.7 miles to the access site on your right.

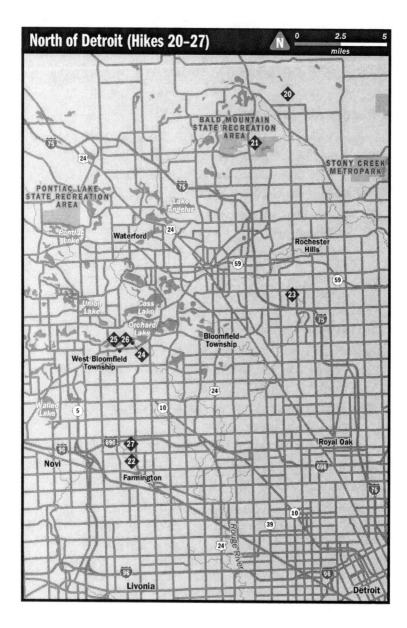

North of Detroit

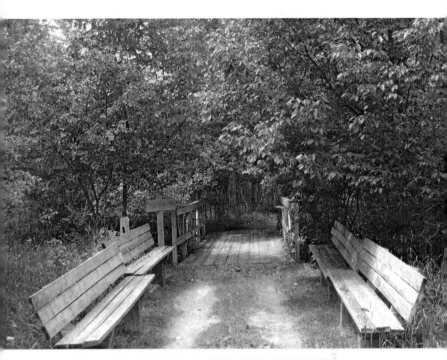

A RESTFUL SPOT AT THE LLOYD A. STAGE NATURE CENTER IN TROY

20 # Bald Mountain State Recreation Area:
North Unit Trails

SCENERY: ★ ★ ★ ★
TRAIL CONDITION: ★ ★ ★ ★ ★
CHILDREN: ★ ★
DIFFICULTY: ★ ★ ★
SOLITUDE: ★ ★ ★

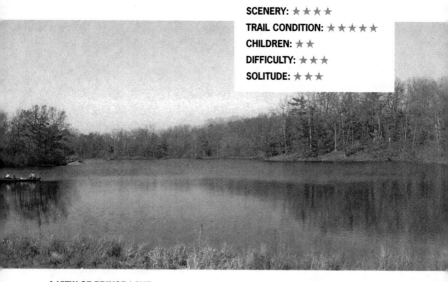

A VIEW OF PRINCE LAKE

GPS TRAILHEAD COORDINATES: N42° 46.995' W83° 11.841'

DISTANCE & CONFIGURATION: 7-mile loop

HIKING TIME: About 3 hours

HIGHLIGHTS: Rolling woodlands, lakes, wetlands

ELEVATION: 970 feet at trailhead, with no significant rise

ACCESS: Daily, 8 a.m.–10 p.m.; $10 annual recreation passport per vehicle

MAPS: At the trailhead and **michigan.gov/dnr**

FACILITIES: None

WHEELCHAIR ACCESS: None

COMMENTS: Portions of the trail cross through areas of the park open to seasonal hunting. Wear an orange vest or jacket during hunting season. It's best to avoid the trail during firearms season for deer in mid- to late November. The trail is extremely popular with bicyclists.

CONTACTS: 248-693-6767; **michigan.gov/dnr**

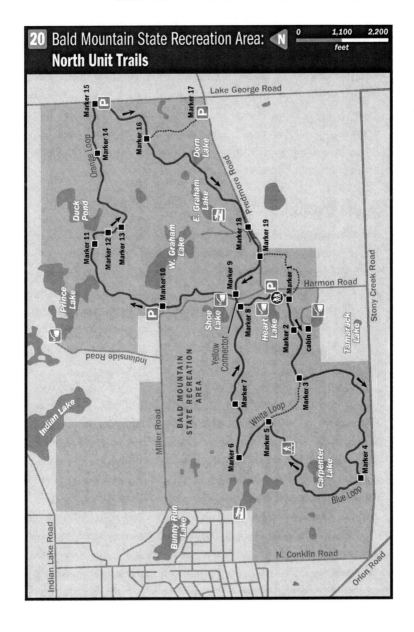

20 Bald Mountain State Recreation Area: **N** North Unit Trails

0   1,100   2,200
feet

Overview

The North Unit Trails of Bald Mountain State Recreation Area traverse some of the hilliest and steepest terrain in southeast Michigan. This portion of the park is thick with hardwood forests and is home to about a dozen lakes, as well as tamarack and cedar swamps. This is one of the region's most scenic networks of trails (see page 135 for another hiking option here). It is especially beautiful from late September to mid-October when the leaves are turning colors.

Route Details

Bald Mountain State Recreation Area in northeast Oakland County offers something for every outdoor enthusiast, from hikers to mountain bikers and anglers to campers. The 4,637-acre park is home to more than 15 miles of marked trails, and most of them lie in the park's North Unit. The trails in the North Unit are the best, looping around several lakes and traversing rugged, thickly wooded terrain. These woods are home to all kinds of wildlife, including white-tailed deer, rabbits, squirrels, and raccoons.

Here I am describing a combination of the network of trails that generally follows the outer loop in the North Unit. Some trails simply serve as loop connectors. Hikers can follow any of the loops or connectors to make their own treks. The trails range in distance from the 0.1-mile Yellow Connector to the 3.6-mile Orange Loop. The latter loops in and around seven lakes. The route described here includes the Orange, Blue, and White loops to create a 7-mile trek, and it passes near most of the lakes in the North Unit.

Begin at the White Loop trailhead off Harmon Road. A small dirt parking lot is on the east side of the road just as it intersects with Predmore Road. The trail begins at the southern end of the parking lot; you'll see wetlands and Heart Lake on your right and Harmon Road on your left. The trail immediately slips into thick woods and narrows as it heads south and then southwest toward markers 2 and 3. This stretch is part of the 2.1-mile White Loop. Hikers will skip a stretch of the White Loop to join the Blue Loop at Marker 3. The Blue Loop rejoins the White Loop at Marker 5. Marker 2 is less than 0.3 miles from the trailhead and stands at an intersection. Swing right, heading due west to Marker 3, about 0.1 mile ahead.

At marker 3, swing left, heading south and southwest to marker 4, on the Blue Loop, which circles around Carpenter Lake. At marker 4, continue straight, heading west. This lovely stretch passes majestic maple trees and towering pines. If you haven't noticed the pine needles littering the trail, you should be able to smell their fragrance. Around the 1.5-mile mark, the trail crosses a small bridge over a creek and then along a boardwalk through wetlands.

At about the 1.8-mile spot, marker 5 stands at the junction of the Blue and White loops. Swing left, heading northwest to marker 6, with wetlands on your left. At marker 6, swing right, heading east and continuing on the White Loop. Again, the landscape is a mix of woods, wetlands, and open fields en route to markers 7 and 8. Marker 8 stands just before Harmon Road at the southern end of Shoe Lake. You should reach this junction around the 2.5-mile mark. Marker 9 stands on the opposite side of the road.

The 0.1-mile Yellow Connector binds the network of trails on the west side of Harmon Road to those on the east side. At marker 9, turn left, heading northeast and then north along the Orange Loop. This section is more open and rises above Harmon Road, which runs parallel to the trail for a long stretch. Marker 10 lies just north of Miller Road and trail access parking.

Prince Lake will come into view on your left as the trail reaches marker 11. Turn right at the T-intersection and continue east. Wetlands and Duck Pond will be visible on your left as you reach marker 12. The next marker, 13, is only 0.1 mile ahead. Continue heading east to markers 14 and 15. When you reach marker 15, you'll see a bench and another trail access point with parking on Lake George Road. Bear right, heading south and then southwest to marker 16. Continue straight at marker 16. The spur on your left leads to marker 17, another trail access spot with parking. Expect stretches of the trail to be wet and muddy as you pass between Dorn Lake and East Graham Lake, between markers 16 and 18. The trail narrows through wetlands and continues on a bridge through wetlands after marker 18. Continue straight at marker 19 as you head back to marker 9, to the Yellow Connector. Cross Harmon Road to marker 8. Turn left and head south back to the trailhead.

Nearby Attractions

In the fall, Upland Hills Farm, about 10 miles northeast of Bald Mountain, complements a colorful hike in the woods. The farm's Harvest Festival in October offers hayrides, pumpkin picking, cow milking, and cider and doughnuts. The area, too, is home to a variety of entertainment venues, including DTE Energy Theater, Meadowbrook Music Hall, Meadowbrook Theater, and the Palace at Auburn Hills.

Directions

From Detroit, take I-75 north about 30 miles to Exit 81, M-24 north, toward Lapeer. Follow M-24 north about 7 miles to Atwater Street. Turn right and follow about 0.5 miles to Orion Road. Turn right. Go another 0.5 miles and turn left onto Stoney Creek Road. Turn left on Harmon Road. The trailhead parking lot will be on the left-hand side about 0.5 miles north at the intersection with Predmore Road.

From Ann Arbor, take US 23 north to M-14 toward Plymouth. Go about 15 miles and merge onto I-275 north. Follow it 6 miles to I-696 east toward Port Huron, then to I-75 north toward Flint, Exit 81, M-24 north. Go about 7 miles. Turn right on Atwater Street. Go about 0.5 miles and turn right on Orion Road. Go another 0.5 miles and turn left onto Stoney Creek Road, then left on Harmon Road. The trailhead parking lot will be on the left-hand side about 0.5 miles north at the intersection with Predmore Road.

21 Bald Mountain Recreation Area:
Red Loop Trail

SCENERY: ★ ★ ★
TRAIL CONDITION: ★ ★
CHILDREN: ★ ★ ★
DIFFICULTY: ★ ★
SOLITUDE: ★ ★ ★

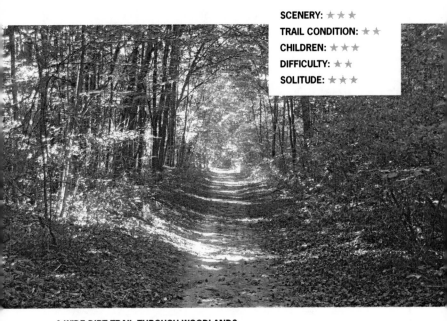

A WIDE DIRT TRAIL THROUGH WOODLANDS

GPS TRAILHEAD COORDINATES: N42° 44.569' W83° 14.104'

DISTANCE & CONFIGURATION: 4.5 miles of connecting loops

HIKING TIME: About 2 hours or less

HIGHLIGHTS: Woodlands, fields, swamps

ELEVATION: 974 feet at trailhead, with no significant rise

ACCESS: Daily, 8 a.m.–10 p.m.; $10 annual recreation passport per vehicle

MAPS: At the park office on Greenshield Road and **michigan.gov/dnr**

FACILITIES: None

WHEELCHAIR ACCESS: None

COMMENTS: The recreation area is open to hunting annually from September 15 to March 31. Mountain biking is permitted on the trail.

CONTACTS: 248-693-6767; **michigan.gov/dnr**

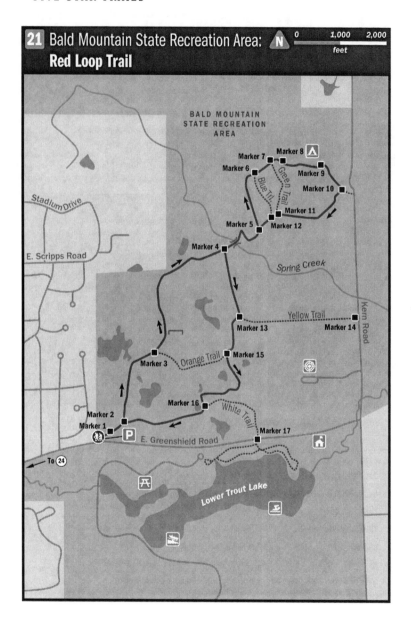

Overview

The Red Loop is the gentler of the two major trail networks at the Bald Mountain State Recreation Area in northern Oakland County and passes mostly through hilly woodlands thick with maples and oaks and laced with wetlands. The trail passes through areas open to hunting, which is especially a concern during firearms season for deer. Wear an orange vest or avoid the trail during mid- to late November.

Route Details

Despite its location in one of southeast Michigan's hilliest regions, the Red Loop is largely gentle and mostly flat. For sure, the trail dips occasionally along its 3.7-mile length, but there's nothing particularly strenuous. And along the hilliest stretches of the southern section of the 4,637-acre park, the trail manages either to follow the crest of a hill or cut along its side.

The main trailhead for the Red Loop is located at the edge of a dirt parking lot on the north side of Greenshield Road, about 0.5 miles east of Lapeer Road (M-24). The trail, however, is also accessible from a second dirt parking lot about 1 mile farther down the road near the park headquarters. From that trailhead, the 0.4-mile White Trail connects to the Red Loop. A series of smaller trails, all named by colors, dissect the Red Trail, creating smaller loops. The White and Yellow trails are linear and connect to parking areas.

From the main Red Loop trailhead, follow the narrow dirt trail, its shoulders mowed on both sides. You will walk through a field, passing an antiquated trail identification system: it is simply a signpost with the intersection marked by a number at its top and an arrow pointing the way to the next numbered intersection. Houses remain visible through the tree line to the west, and the trail descends gently, reaching a cluster of trees after about 500 feet. At this juncture, you can turn in either direction to follow the Red Loop.

To follow the sequence of trail intersections in order, swing left and continue north-northeast. You'll reach marker 2 at the 0.1-mile mark. From here, the fields become thicker with trees on both sides and you'll notice a series of large anthills on your left. The dirt trail becomes wider, and ponds are visible through the tree line on your left. At about 0.4 miles, you reach marker 3. Bear left. The Orange Trail will be on your right and reconnects with the Red Loop about 0.7 miles east.

The stretch between markers 3 and 4 is among the longest between markers—about 0.5 miles. The terrain is largely wooded, and a bench near the 0.5-mile mark sits under three towering oak trees. Be aware that you are ultimately heading north-northeast. When you come to an unmarked T-intersection, around the 0.7-mile mark, swing right. (Heading the opposite direction leads to the edge of a high school and a network of unmarked trails.)

From the 0.7-mile mark, the trail rises, and ponds are visible through trees. Another trail intersects this stretch, but you should continue northeast, bearing right. The trail descends to marker 4, near the 1-mile mark. Veer left toward marker 5, crossing a natural bridge over Spring Creek and continuing northeast. The trail ascends, passing swamps and steep slopes on either side of the trail, but flattens as it approaches marker 5, near the 1.3-mile mark.

Swing left, heading northwest to marker 6, about 0.2 miles ahead. You'll pass another swamp on your right, and the trail slopes downward, passing through scattered pines. Reach marker 6 at about 1.4 miles. Swing left; the trail immediately drops, and the next pair of markers, 7 and 8, are within 0.1 mile of each other.

Heading east toward marker 9, you will note that the trail flattens and widens, resembling an old country road. You'll find marker 9 near the 1.7-mile mark, on your right. A spur at marker 10 simply leads east to Kern Road. Ignore that and continue southwest, passing markers 11 and 12 at the intersections of the Green and Blue trails, respectively. You're still heading south-southwest, crossing Spring Creek and then passing along rolling terrain on your way back to marker 4.

From there, swing left, bearing south to marker 13. The trail becomes gentler over the last mile or so but frequently passes swamps and wetlands en route to the trailhead. Don't be surprised—or alarmed—to hear gunshots in the distance; the park shooting range is to the east, off Kern Road.

At about the 3-mile mark, the trail intersects with the White Trail, which leads to the parking lot across from the park office. Swing right and continue west to marker 2 and go about 0.7 miles to return to the trailhead.

Nearby Attractions

Northern Oakland County is home to several parks for hiking and other outdoor activities. About 10 miles northwest of Bald Mountain is Independence Oaks County Park, which boasts some of the county park system's best trails—more than 10 miles of them, and fairly well marked. One of the newest is the 2.2-mile River Loop Trail, which features a boardwalk through wetlands. The 2.3-mile Lakeshore Trail runs along the perimeter of Crooked Lake. The 1.6-mile Springlake Trail covers some of the most rugged terrain in northern Oakland County.

Directions

From Detroit, take I-75 north to Exit 81, Lapeer Road/M-24. Follow M-24 north about 3.4 miles to Greenshield Road. Turn right. The parking lot and trailhead will be about 0.5 miles down on your left.

From Ann Arbor, take US 23 north to M-14, Exit 42, toward Plymouth. Follow M-14 about 14 miles and merge north onto I-275. Follow I-275 about 6 miles to I-696 east. Continue to I-75 north toward Flint. Take Exit 81, Lapeer Road, to M-24 north. Head north about 3.4 miles to Greenshield Road. Turn right. The parking lot and trailhead are on your left, about 0.5 miles down.

Heritage Park: River Trail

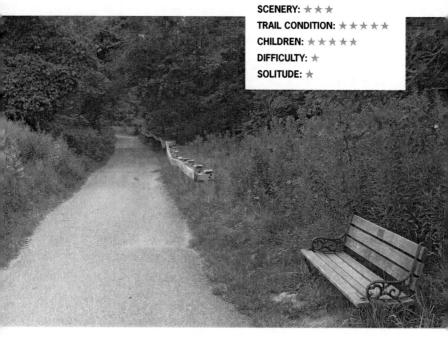

SCENERY: ★ ★ ★
TRAIL CONDITION: ★ ★ ★ ★ ★
CHILDREN: ★ ★ ★ ★ ★
DIFFICULTY: ★
SOLITUDE: ★

A BENCH BECKONS HIKERS TO SIT AND LISTEN TO SONGBIRDS.

GPS TRAILHEAD COORDINATES: N42° 47.589' W83 37.887'

DISTANCE & CONFIGURATION: 1-mile balloon

HIKING TIME: 1 hour or less

HIGHLIGHTS: Woodlands, wetlands, Rouge River

ELEVATION: 795 feet at trailhead, with no significant rise

ACCESS: Daily, 8 a.m.–sunset; no fees or permits required

MAPS: At the trailhead and **fhgov.com**

FACILITIES: Restrooms, picnic areas, visitor center, nature center

WHEELCHAIR ACCESS: The beginning of the trail is paved and wheelchair accessible.

COMMENTS: Pets prohibited; busy park. During early June, I found the trail muddy in long stretches and heavy with black flies. The trails are open year-round but can become unpassable during heavy snow and ice in winter or because of mud during the spring.

CONTACTS: 248-473-1800; **fhgov.com**

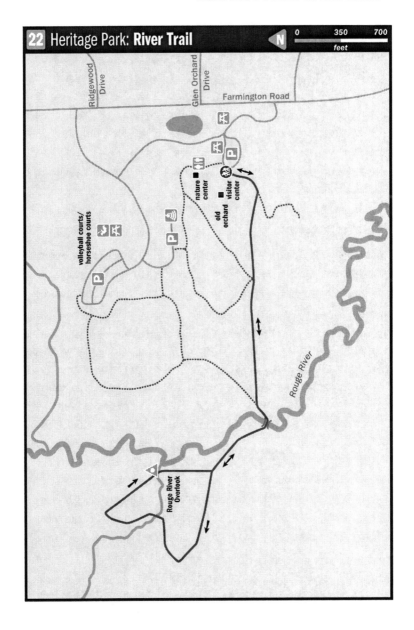

Overview

Heritage Park provides a glimpse of what much of suburban Detroit was like before sprawl and development took place in the mid- to late 20th century. The park has 4.5 miles of trails that traverse gentle hills, meadows, wetlands, and forests of hardwood trees. One of the region's most famous waterways, the Rouge River, meanders through the park's lowlands. The park is home to a visitor center, a pond, an amphitheater, horseshoe courts, sand volleyball courts, playgrounds, and a nature center.

Route Details

Finding a decent hiking trail in a city park seems like an oxymoron. But the River Trail in Farmington Hills's Heritage Park manages to be a worthy route as it weaves its way far from the well-manicured expanse and deep into the woods.

The River Trail begins at the edge of a parking lot and the lovely grounds of the former Spicer estate. The English country house that serves as the visitor center was built in 1926 for an attorney and his wife. The husband passed away before ever having the opportunity to live in the manse, and the wife gave the home to the Spicer family when the couple married. The Spicers created a 200-acre farm; the owner referred to the tract as "the only unspoiled place in Farmington Hills." It may very well still be. Today, of course, the estate is Heritage Park, and the house is considered the park's crown jewel.

The 211-acre site features ten trails, varying in length from about 100 yards to the 1-mile-long River Trail, probably the most scenic of them all. All of the trails are connected, creating a 4.5-mile network; most of them are short, linear paths leading to others. To do them all would require backtracking.

Some of the trails are paved and, for the most part, are named after the park's geographical features. The Orchard Trail, for instance, crosses the estate's former orchard. The Meadow Trail meanders through open fields. The Estate and Spicer trails circle the Spicer house. Connecting directly to the River Trail are the Orchard, Valley, Meadow, and River View trails. (Hike them all and you'll add 1 mile to the described route.)

The River Trail starts at the edge of the parking lot in front of the visitor center as a paved path—a deceptive beginning to the trail's eventual form. Enjoy a pleasant stroll along the paved path through fields brimming with wildflowers and thick brush. Once the River Trail crosses the Orchard Trail, the pavement yields to dirt and stone, and the trail takes you through a marshy area teeming with cattails and reeds. Dead trees dot the surface of the marsh, and thick brush frames the wetlands.

The first impression is that this is a typical southeastern Michigan landscape, with open meadows, gentle hills, wetlands, and hardwood forests. Wildflowers flourish along the gentle trail in the warmer months, and you will notice benches and trash bins along the way.

As the trail continues due west, the woods become thicker, and the noise from the parking lot and park facilities fades. Stand still, and you can hear familiar birds—such as warblers, chickadees, nuthatches, and cardinals—chirping away and the wind rustling through the leaves. In the spring and fall, the chirping is even louder as migrant birds rest around the marsh area bordering the southern stretch of the trail. Such revelry will be short-lived, however; the trail is busy with senior citizens, Scouts, and other groups out for a leisurely stroll.

The trail crosses a small bridge over the Rouge River and winds its way through the woods. At a fork, bear left and follow a loop as it rounds through the forest. This balloon crosses a series of gentle hills common in parts of southeast Michigan. As you make your way around the balloon, you'll come across a scenic view of the meandering Rouge River. Amazingly, I enjoyed this spot and the loop without the company of others. A wood fence guards the bluff, and trees hang over the river. From the overlook, continue on the trail until you close the loop. From here, retrace your route to the parking lot.

Nearby Activities

Just 1 mile north of Farmington Road, Woodland Hills Nature Park offers a quieter, more rustic hiking experience. A network of trails winds through one of the last vestiges of beech-maple forest in the area. An expansive swath of trees in the park's center includes mature maple, black cherry, and oak trees, as well as nesting areas for great horned and screech owls and red-tailed hawks. The park attracts hikers, bird-watchers, and photographers.

Directions

From Detroit, take US 10 (Lodge Freeway) north to I-696 west, then to the Orchard Lake Road, Exit 42. Turn left and continue about 0.7 miles to 11 Mile Road. Turn right and continue 1 mile to Farmington Road. Turn left. The entrance to Heritage Park is 0.4 miles south on your right.

From Ann Arbor, take US 23 north to M-14 east. Follow M-14 about 14 miles to I-275 north. Take I-275 north about 6 miles to I-696 east. Take Orchard Lake Road, Exit 42. Turn right and drive 0.7 miles to 11 Mile Road. Turn right on 11 Mile Road and go about 1 mile to Farmington Road. Turn left on Farmington Road; the park entrance is 0.4 miles on your right.

23 Lloyd A. Stage Nature Center Loops

SCENERY: ★ ★ ★
TRAIL CONDITION: ★ ★ ★ ★ ★
CHILDREN: ★ ★ ★ ★
DIFFICULTY: ★
SOLITUDE: ★ ★ ★

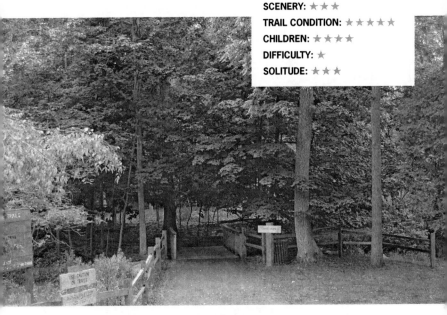

A BRIDGE OVER THE NORTH BRANCH OF THE ROUGE RIVER

GPS TRAILHEAD COORDINATES: N42° 36.976' W83° 11.535'

DISTANCE & CONFIGURATION: 1.4 miles of connecting loops

HIKING TIME: About 1 hour

HIGHLIGHTS: Woodlands, meadows, marshland

ELEVATION: 662 feet at trailhead, with no significant rise

ACCESS: Tuesday–Saturday, 8:30 a.m.–4:30 p.m.; Sunday, noon–5 p.m. $3, adults; $2, children ages 6–17; free, children under age 6

MAPS: At the nature center

FACILITIES: Restrooms, gift shop, library, nature center

WHEELCHAIR ACCESS: Yes, the nature center and a small portion outside the nature center are paved; however, the trails are easily navigable with wheelchairs.

COMMENTS: No pets, bicycles, jogging, or cross-country skiing allowed.

CONTACTS: 248-524-3567; **troymi.gov/parksrec/naturecenter**

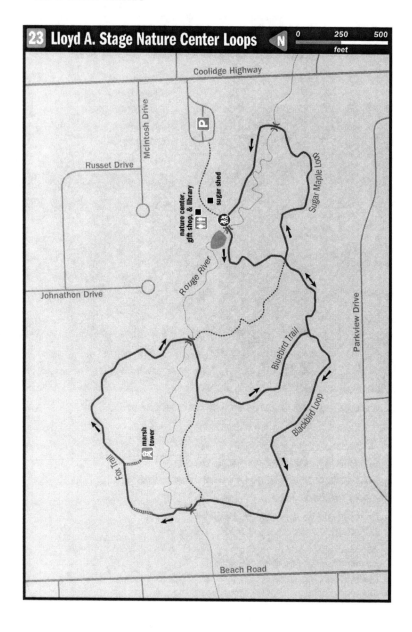

23 Lloyd A. Stage Nature Center Loops

N

0   250   500
feet

Coolidge Highway

McIntosh Drive

Russet Drive

sugar shed

nature center,
gift shop, & library

Rouge River

Sugar Maple Loop

Johnathon Drive

Bluebird Trail

Blackbird Loop

Parkview Drive

Fox Trail

marsh
tower

Beach Road

Overview

At the Lloyd A. Stage Nature Center at the northern edge of Troy, gentle trails interlace through old- and new-growth forests and across a narrow stream, the headwaters of the north branch of the Rouge River. Small fields and meadows occasionally interrupt the wooded trails, and a boardwalk leads to a small observation tower in a marsh, rich with trees, shrubs, and other vegetation.

Route Details

The Lloyd A. Stage Nature Center boasts just 1.6 miles of trails amid wet forests, sedge meadows, and cattail marshes, but even the most ardent hiker would find these woods pleasant and a welcome respite from the surrounding housing developments in the "City of Tomorrow . . . Today." The trails are well maintained, well marked, and easy to follow. And despite their brevity, the trails cover a remarkably diverse terrain in a small area. The nature center property, formerly part of a farm and private homes, encompasses just 100 acres.

Four trails make up the loops: Blackbird, Sugar Maple, Fox, and Bluebird. The Blackbird Loop and Sugar Maple Loop are the longest, at 0.7 and 0.4 miles, respectively. The Fox Trail forms a half loop beyond the Blackbird Loop and measures just 0.4 miles. The smallest of the trails, the Bluebird Trail, dissects the Blackbird Loop and is just over 0.1 mile. Combining the trails creates a 1.4-mile hike.

From the nature center building, follow either of two asphalt paths that lead to the **Sugar Maple Loop**; one heads southwest toward a pond and the Rouge River, and the other goes southeast.

The trailhead is about 30 feet from the nature center building, at the beginning of the Sugar Maple Loop. A large wooden sign notes trail names and distances. A small wooden bridge crosses the river; a pond on the right is frequented by Canada geese, ducks, and other waterfowl.

The mulched trail heads southwest and intersects with the **Blackbird Loop** at about 150 feet. Swing right and head west along the Blackbird Loop, walking amid towering new- and old-growth trees. Oak, maple, black cherry, box elder, and hickory trees fill the woods here. Beyond the tree line on the left, houses in a neighboring development are visible.

The **Bluebird Trail** intersects the Blackbird Loop at about the 0.2-mile mark. From here, continue west on the Blackbird Loop along a grassy trail (you'll return to the Bluebird Trail later). A series of dirt steps eases the trek up a slight hill to a pair of benches and a split-rail fence bordering a meadow. The woods become thicker as the Blackbird Loop approaches the **Fox Trail,** at about the 0.4-mile mark.

Don't be surprised to find white-tailed deer grazing in fields or walking through the woods. Wildlife abounds on the premises. Also be on the lookout for wild turkeys, raccoons, opossums, gray foxes, red squirrels, groundhogs, and weasels. You may spot mink and coyotes on the grounds, too.

Here, you can either continue east along the **Blackbird Loop** or swing left along the **Fox Trail** into an expansive marsh. Following the Fox Trail, the path almost immediately crosses the Rouge River and becomes a narrow dirt trail to a series of boardwalks. About the 0.5-mile mark, a boardwalk on your right leads to the Marsh Tower (just 12 steps up to a wooden platform), which offers a panoramic view of the marsh, thick with shrubs and trees. Other than a birdhouse here or there, there are no man-made intrusions.

Back on the **Fox Trail,** the narrow dirt path crosses under a tunnel of low-growth, craggy trees and passes an outdoor classroom before becoming a boardwalk running alongside the Rouge River. After crossing the Rouge, swing right and follow the **Blackbird Loop** west. The **Bluebird Trail** intersects at about the 0.8-mile mark. Head south along that trail, crossing a field and scattered trees to connect to the southern stretch of the **Blackbird Loop.**

Retrace your steps along the Blackbird Loop, walking east, to return to the **Sugar Maple Loop** at about the 1-mile mark. Do not head back to the nature center the way you came, but continue east; you are now hiking another section of the Sugar Maple Loop. The trail passes through a grove of old-growth sugar maples. Sugar maples are the dominant maples here, some a couple hundred years old, but silver and black maples can be spotted, too.

As the trail loops back to the nature center building, you'll pass a sugar shed on your right. The shed is used for maple syrup demonstrations in March. Continuing northwest, you'll end up at the large wooden information sign you passed at the beginning of the hike. The nature center will be on your right.

Nearby Activities

Troy offers the best of both the old and new. One of the region's premier malls, the Somerset Collection, is 4 miles south along Coolidge Road at West Big Beaver Road. The mall boasts upscale shopping at retailers such as Saks Fifth Avenue, Barneys, and Neiman Marcus. Three miles northeast, the Troy Museum and Historic Village tells the story of the city's past as depicted in ten buildings surrounding a village green.

Directions

From Detroit, follow I-75 north about 23 miles, to Exit 74, Adams Road. Turn left onto Adams Road. Turn right on South Boulevard. Drive 1 mile to Coolidge Highway. Turn right on Coolidge Highway. Turn right into the nature center.

From Ann Arbor, take M-14 to I-275, for about 15 miles. Follow I-275 north about 18 miles to Exit 165, I-696 east. Follow I-696 east to I-75 north. Follow I-75 north about 13 miles to Exit 74, Adams Road. Turn left onto Adams. Turn right on South Boulevard. Drive 1 mile to Coolidge Highway. Turn right on Coolidge Highway. Turn right into the nature center.

24

Orchard Lake
Nature Sanctuary

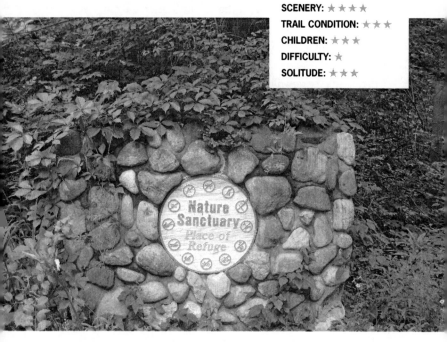

SCENERY: ★ ★ ★ ★
TRAIL CONDITION: ★ ★ ★
CHILDREN: ★ ★ ★
DIFFICULTY: ★
SOLITUDE: ★ ★ ★

A STONE SIGN MARKS A "PLACE OF REFUGE."

GPS TRAILHEAD COORDINATES: N42° 34.450' W83° 22.486'
DISTANCE & CONFIGURATION: 1.6-mile connecting loops
HIKING TIME: About 1 hour or less
HIGHLIGHTS: Lakes, old-growth woods, wetlands
ELEVATION: 1,010 feet at trailhead, with no significant rise
ACCESS: Daily, sunrise–sunset; no fees or permits required
MAPS: Displayed at trailhead
FACILITIES: Primitive restroom and picnic pavilion
WHEELCHAIR ACCESS: None
COMMENTS: No pets or bicycles allowed
CONTACTS: 248-682-2400

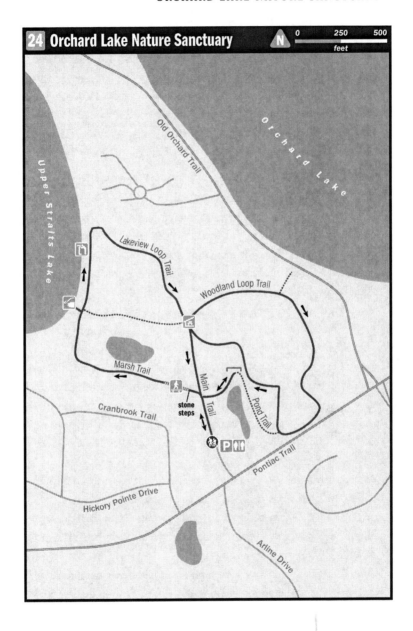

Overview

The sanctuary's Main Trail, Marsh Trail, Lakeview Loop, Woodland Loop, and Pond Trail weave through stately old- and new-growth forests amid the rolling terrain in northwestern Oakland County. The five trails also wind around wetlands and a vernal pond. Snow glories bloom in the spring, blanketing the forest grounds in purple and blue.

Route Details

This 50-acre tract tucked between Orchard Lake and Upper Straits Lake is truly a sanctuary from the commercial hub along Pontiac Trail and the tony subdivisions surrounding the lakes of northwestern Oakland County. The white noise of traffic is ever present in the woods, but the magnificent trees and pines create the illusion of being far away from it all.

You could easily miss the sanctuary if you are traveling in either direction along Pontiac Trail. Only a brown road sign that denotes a nature sanctuary 500 feet away gives any indication that something special is tucked into a patch of woods along this road. Owned by the city of Orchard Lake, the refuge once belonged to the Ward family, lumber barons and stewards of the environment who donated the property to the Cranbrook Educational Community. The city saved the tract from possible development when Cranbrook decided to sell the land in the 1990s.

Start your tranquil quest at the trailhead, at the end of the small gravel parking lot, where a sign marks the sanctuary's approximately 1.6 miles of trails named above. The wide, graveled **Main Trail** connects all four of them, and at major intersections, signs with permanent maps display the trail details.

You may create your own hiking configurations here, and the trails are so gentle that you could walk them more than once on any given outing. The route I followed encompasses the **Main Trail, Marsh Trail, Woodland Loop,** and **Pond Trail**; only a portion of the **Lakeview Loop** is left out of this trek.

Head north from the **Main** trailhead along the wide, graveled trail that connects the small trail network. In early spring, the forest grounds on your right present a carpet of blue and purple, thanks to blooming snow glories.

Swing left onto a trail about 200 feet from your start to follow the **Marsh Trail.** The mulched path narrows and leads down a series of stone steps to a boardwalk that borders the shoreline. While houses remain visible through the tree line up the hill on your left side, the landscape around the marsh is thick with trees, especially maples. Dotting the marsh are stands of dead ash trees—victims of the emerald ash borer.

As the trail winds around the marsh, it rises and intersects with **Lakeview Loop Trail** at about the 0.3-mile mark. A spur on the left leads to a fishing dock, just a short walk away, and offers a nice view of Upper Straits Lake, which, as you might have expected, is ringed with houses.

Returning to the intersection, swing left along the rising trail, climbing above Upper Straits Lake, slightly visible through the trees. A wooden observation deck juts out into the lake along this stretch.

The **Lakeview Loop Trail** intersects with the **Main Trail** and the **Woodland Loop Trail** at about the 0.5-mile point. Boulders line the trails, marking the intersection. As the **Lakeview Loop Trail** spills onto the **Main Trail,** take a hard left onto the **Woodland Loop Trail,** passing a picnic pavilion on your right. The pavilion was once part of Cranbrook's outdoor science classroom. This trail loops through an old-growth forest, rich with towering oaks, some 250–300 years old, and passes briefly through a field before returning to the forest. Other tree varieties share the forest with magnificent oaks. They include hickories, maples, hemlocks, and white pines.

The road and passing traffic become visible for a brief stretch, but the trail quickly winds back into the woods, passing a bench at the 0.6-mile mark.

A spur on the left leads to the road. The next intersection occurs at the 0.8-mile mark; swing right and follow it past a pond on your left. The trail eases onto the **Main Trail.** At this juncture, you're on the opposite side of the pavilion you passed at the beginning of the trail, and you'll find a 5- to 6-acre prairie directly in front of you. Turn left and head back to the trailhead.

At the 1-mile mark, the Pond Trail on your left leads to a vernal pond. The path is only about 0.1 mile long but connects to the Main Trail. From here, continue along the Woodland Loop Trail before reconnecting with the Main Trail near the picnic pavilion. Swing left and head south back toward the trailhead. I swung left at the intersection with the Pond Trail and walked to the vernal pond (you'll find a bench overlooking the pond) and then retraced my steps back to the Main Trail. Swing left again; the trailhead is directly ahead. While this hike is short, the trails pass through beautiful thick woods and around wetlands, as well as offer scenic lake views. The Orchard Lake Nature Sanctuary is such an inviting retreat—don't be surprised if you're tempted to walk it again and again.

Nearby Attractions

Just down Orchard Lake Road are the West Bloomfield Woods Nature Preserve (see page 160) and the West Bloomfield Trail (see page 155).

Directions

From Detroit, take the Lodge Freeway, M-10, north about 20 miles to Orchard Lake Road. Turn right on Orchard Lake Road and follow it about 3.5 miles to Pontiac Trail. Turn left on Pontiac Trail. The nature sanctuary is about 0.8 miles farther along on the left-hand side.

From Ann Arbor, follow M-14 east to I-275. Merge onto I-275 and go north about 6 miles to M-5 north/I-696, Exit 165, toward Grand River Avenue/Port Huron. Take the M-5 north exit on the left. Drive about 5 miles to Pontiac Trail. Turn right onto Pontiac Trail and continue about 4 miles to the nature sanctuary, which will be on your left.

25

West Bloomfield Trail

SCENERY: ★ ★ ★
TRAIL CONDITION: ★ ★ ★ ★ ★
CHILDREN: ★ ★ ★ ★ ★
DIFFICULTY: ★
SOLITUDE: ★

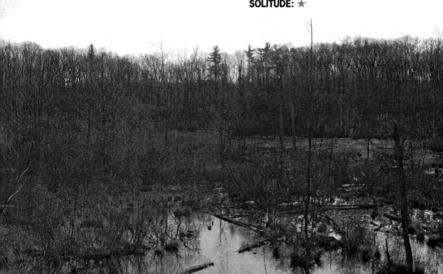

EXPANSIVE WETLANDS ALONG THE WEST BLOOMFIELD TRAIL

GPS TRAILHEAD COORDINATES: N42° 34.075' W83° 23.585'
DISTANCE & CONFIGURATION: 4.3-mile point-to-point with shuttle
HIKING TIME: About 2 hours
HIGHLIGHTS: Wetlands, woodlands, lakes
ELEVATION: 1,014 feet, with no significant rise
ACCESS: Daily, 8 a.m.–sunset; no fees or permits required
MAPS: At the trailhead and **westbloomfieldparks.org**
FACILITIES: Primitive restrooms, picnic area
WHEELCHAIR ACCESS: Yes
COMMENTS: The trail is open to bicyclists and inline skaters.
CONTACTS: 248-451-1900; **westbloomfieldparks.org**

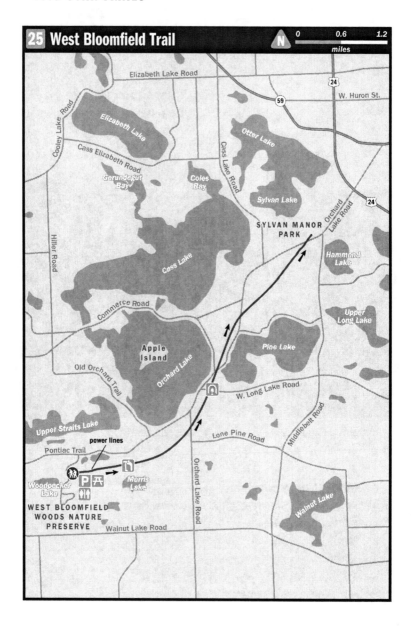

Overview

The former right-of-way of an early Michigan railroad today is a favorite recreation path stretching from the West Bloomfield Woods Nature Preserve to Sylvan Manor Park. Along its 4.3-mile route, the gentle paved trail passes through wetlands and thin woodlands and around lakes. Interpretive signs explain various habitats. While the trail skirts subdivisions and weaves near some busy intersections, it remains a pleasant walk, especially in the spring and fall.

Route Details

The West Bloomfield Trail is a 28-acre linear park that begins just off the east side of a parking lot shared with the West Bloomfield Woods Nature Preserve, a 162-acre tract that is home to old-growth forests, carpets of springtime wildflowers, and wildlife, and is frequented by more than 100 species of birds.

The West Bloomfield Trail itself, on the other hand, passes through residential and commercial areas, but still manages to touch upon some of the region's diverse habitats and flora. While far less rustic than its counterpart, it's no less interesting or less worthy of exploration.

From the trailhead, you will walk east-northeast to Sylvan Manor Park, passing along woods on your right and power lines on your left. Among the first natural habitats the trail crosses are vernal ponds. They're home to wood frogs, spring peepers, nonpoisonous snakes, and salamanders, which make their way to the ponds in the spring to mate.

Around the 0.4-mile mark, an observation deck with a telescope offers an up-close glimpse of wetlands on your right. More than 50 great blue herons nest in the wooded wetlands, and the best time to see them is late March–June. Careful observers might also spot northern water snakes sunning on logs, rare Blanding's turtles, muskrats, mink, wood ducks, or even deer or coyotes along its edges.

Around the 0.5-mile mark, the trail crosses a subdivision road and passes houses and more wetlands on your left. The next crossing is at Orchard Lake Road, a little more than 1 mile ahead. On the way, the trail passes more houses and wetlands. Shagbark hickory trees are common along this stretch, and it's possible to spot red foxes and eastern coyotes along the trail in quieter hours.

After Orchard Lake Road, the trail passes near shopping centers and then runs through a tunnel under Long Lake Road just before it cuts through the narrow area between Orchard and Pine lakes. An interpretive sign points out Apple Island in Orchard Lake. Now owned by the West Bloomfield Schools, the island has a storied past: white settlers colonized the island, and Chief Pontiac of the Ottawa tribe held council there. Some believe it was here that he planned his attack on Fort Detroit. Today, the island is used as an educational nature center.

Between Pine and Orchard lakes, the trail crosses through small wetlands. Be on the lookout for migrant birds. Among the most common are red-winged blackbirds. You'll also spot Canada geese and mute swans. Beyond Pine Lake, look for majestic oaks in a field on the eastern side of the trail. They're frequent perches for red-tailed hawks. As the trail continues north-northeast, after crossing Pine Lake and Commerce roads, thickets become more pronounced. This stretch is a haven for robins, cardinals, chickadees, and warblers. Despite being surrounded by homes and businesses along stretches, don't be surprised to find white-tailed deer crossing or grazing near more isolated spots. The trail ends at Sylvan Manor Park.

From here, retrace your steps back to the starting point. Or, to avoid the hike back, have friends join you and leave one vehicle at the Sylvan Manor Park lot and one at the lot at the West Bloomfield trailhead. From this point, the trail continues as the Clinton River Trail, which follows another abandoned rail line from Sylvan Park all the way to Rochester, about 16 miles northeast. The trail passes through Rochester and meets the Macomb Orchard Trail at Dequindre Road.

Nearby Attractions

The Holocaust Memorial Center Zekelman Family Campus, the country's first freestanding Holocaust museum, is in West Bloomfield on Orchard Lake Road, about 7 miles south of the trail. Here, visitors can explore Jewish heritage, the planned extermination of Jews by the Nazis during World War II, and the role of the many who tried to save Jews. The center includes a gift shop and library and is closed on Jewish holidays and most legal holidays.

Directions

From Detroit, take I-75 north to I-696 west. Take I-696 west to the Orchard Lake Road, Exit 42. Turn right and drive about 6 miles to Pontiac Trail. Turn left and continue about 1.5 miles to Arrowhead Road. Turn left and go about 0.5 miles to the preserve entrance on the left. The trailhead is just off the parking lot.

From Ann Arbor, take US 23 north to M-14 east. Follow M-14 about 14 miles to I-275 north. Take I-275 north about 6 miles to I-696 east. Take Orchard Lake Road, Exit 42. Turn left and go about 6 miles to Pontiac Trail. Turn left and continue about 1.5 miles to Arrowhead Road. Turn left. The park entrance is about 0.5 miles ahead on the left. The trailhead is just off the parking lot.

26 # West Bloomfield Woods Nature Preserve

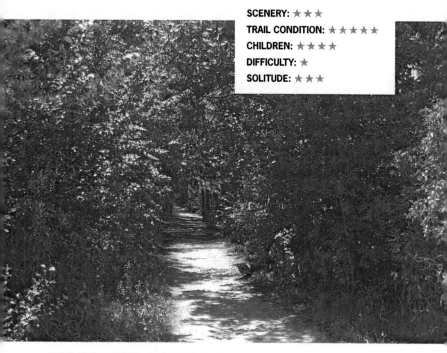

SCENERY: ★ ★ ★
TRAIL CONDITION: ★ ★ ★ ★ ★
CHILDREN: ★ ★ ★ ★
DIFFICULTY: ★
SOLITUDE: ★ ★ ★

THICK FOLIAGE HIDES SURROUNDING HOUSING DEVELOPMENTS.

GPS TRAILHEAD COORDINATES: N42° 56.789' W83° 39.317'
DISTANCE & CONFIGURATION: 2.5-mile balloon
HIKING TIME: About 1 hour
HIGHLIGHTS: Woodlands, wetlands, wildflowers
ELEVATION: 1,014 feet at the trailhead, with no significant rise
ACCESS: Daily, 8 a.m.–sunset; no fees or permits required
MAPS: At trailhead and **westbloomfieldparks.org**
FACILITIES: Restrooms, picnic areas
WHEELCHAIR ACCESS: Yes, for 0.5 miles of the trail
COMMENTS: Pets must be kept on 6-foot leash.
CONTACTS: 248-738-2500; **westbloomfieldparks.org**

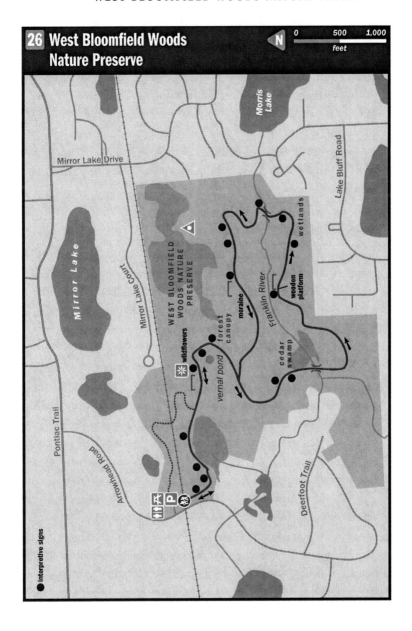

Overview

Tucked away off a busy stretch of Pontiac Trail in northern Oakland County, the West Bloomfield Woods Nature Preserve offers a tranquil escape from the surrounding suburbia. The gentle 2.5-mile trail meanders through mature woods of oaks, hickory, and wild dogwoods and around wetlands, swamps, ponds, and a stretch of the Franklin River (a branch of the Rouge River). Wild and domestic flowers—wild geraniums, marsh marigolds, and trilliums—flood the woodland floor in the spring.

Route Details

The West Bloomfield Woods Nature Preserve trail begins as a wide gravel path just south of the kiosk in the parking lot at the preserve's entrance. Another trail, the West Bloomfield Trail (see page 155), is a 28-acre linear park that runs through West Bloomfield, Orchard Lake, Keego Harbor, and Sylvan Lake, eventually connecting to the Clinton River and Macomb Orchard trails—far to the east.

The nature preserve trail cuts immediately into the forest, covering hikers under a thick canopy of foliage. The sounds of the suburbs—lawn mowers, cars, and trucks—are never far away, and a residential street is initially visible along the trail's western edge.

Still, 16 interpretative signs dot the course of the trail, explaining flora, fauna, and wetlands, and some of the human history, as well as explaining how glaciers shaped the region.

The first three signs come almost immediately, helping hikers slow down and observe the scenery. One points out a 300-year-old oak tree, a reminder of how the county of Oaks earned its name.

In spring the forest floor is a carpet of colors—yellow, pink, purple, and blue—thanks to thousands of blooming wildflowers: trout lilies, hepatica, and spring beauties, to name a few. Some are old-world flowers planted by the Ward family, former owners of the preserve. These early owners of the land planted narcissus and scilla bulbs, the blue in the forest carpet, from the Netherlands. One of the Wards aptly described the tract as "150 acres of wild and rugged country."

"The woods are for walking and for that you are welcome," reads a sign where an entrance gate to the woods once stood. Soon after, an interpretive sign describes how the hollow of a tree is used as a home for various wildlife, including raccoons, squirrels, and smaller creatures such as mice and toads. Through the trees you can see wetlands, and in spring you'll hear a cacophony of chorus frogs, spring peepers, and wood frogs. In the warmer months, it's common to see northern water snakes and painted turtles sunning themselves on downed trees. These woods, too, are home to more than 100 species of birds: brown creepers, yellow warblers, northern orioles, and great horned owls. Benches along the trail entice hikers to stop, look, and listen.

After passing interpretative sign 6, the trail flattens and the woods become thin, offering hikers a broader view of the lush landscape. At the fork, veer to the right as the red arrow on the post indicates. In the spring and early summer, small vernal ponds are visible through the trees. After crossing a bridge over a creek, the trail runs along a creek, often dry in summer months. Occasionally, you can spot white pines amid the hardwoods.

Another bench is located at interpretative sign 10, where a wooden platform affords a scenic view of the Franklin River and its floodplain. Marsh marigolds, wild irises, and willows blanket the banks. The river is generally nothing more than a trickle during the dry summer months but gushes with cold, swiftly moving water in early spring.

At the next interpretative sign, downed trees and stumps litter the wetlands. From here, the trail rises slightly and a long wooden bridge crosses the Franklin River. Scattered houses can be seen through the woods at the preserve's eastern edge. The woods are thick with dead trees, and woodpeckers are common. Look (or listen) for downy, hairy, and red-headed species.

As the trail heads westward, it passes through more wetlands. Along the trail, witch hazel shrubs burst, typically in November, with tiny yellow flowers. And over the ridge beyond interpretative sign 15 lie the nests of some 100 great blue herons. The spot is not accessible from the preserve nature trail, however; to get there, use the trail network east of the Arrowhead Road parking lot.

Continue west to marker 16. At the fork, turn right and head back to the starting point, retracing your steps to the trailhead.

Nearby Activities

The nature preserve is the western trailhead of the West Bloomfield Trail Network (see page 155), a 4.3-mile rails-to-trails project that meanders through wildflowers, wetlands, woodlands, suburban neighborhoods, and business districts. The trail draws all kinds of outdoor enthusiasts—hikers, bikers, inline skaters, and cross-country skiers—as well as families out for a stroll along a pleasant route.

Directions

From Detroit, take I-75 north I-696 west. Take I-696 west to the Orchard Lake Road, Exit 42. Turn right and drive about 6 miles to Pontiac Trail. Turn left and continue about 1.5 miles to Arrowhead Road. Turn left and go about 0.5 miles to the preserve entrance on the left. The trailhead is just off the parking lot.

From Ann Arbor, take US 23 north to M-14 east. Follow M-14 about 14 miles to I-275 north. Take I-275 north about 6 miles to I-696 east. Take Orchard Lake Road, Exit 42. Turn left and go about 6 miles to Pontiac Trail. Turn left and continue about 1.5 miles to Arrowhead Road. Turn left. The park entrance is about 0.5 miles ahead on the left. The trailhead is just off the parking lot.

Woodland Hills

SCENERY: ★ ★ ★
TRAIL CONDITION: ★ ★ ★ ★
CHILDREN: ★ ★ ★
DIFFICULTY: ★
SOLITUDE: ★ ★ ★

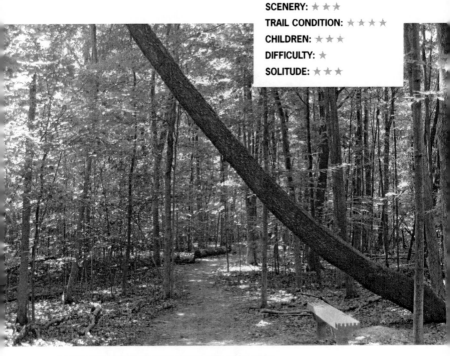

A TREE ARCHES ACROSS A HEAVILY WOODED TRAIL.

GPS TRAILHEAD COORDINATES: N42° 29.560' W83° 22.700'
DISTANCE & CONFIGURATION: 1.7 miles of connecting trails
HIKING TIME: About 1 hour
HIGHLIGHTS: Woodlands, wetlands, Rouge River tributary
ELEVATION: 843 feet at trailhead, with no significant rise
ACCESS: Daily, 8 a.m.–sunset; no fees or permits required
MAPS: At the trailhead
FACILITIES: None
WHEELCHAIR ACCESS: None
COMMENTS: Pets prohibited.
CONTACTS: 248-473-1800; ci.farmington-hills.mi.us

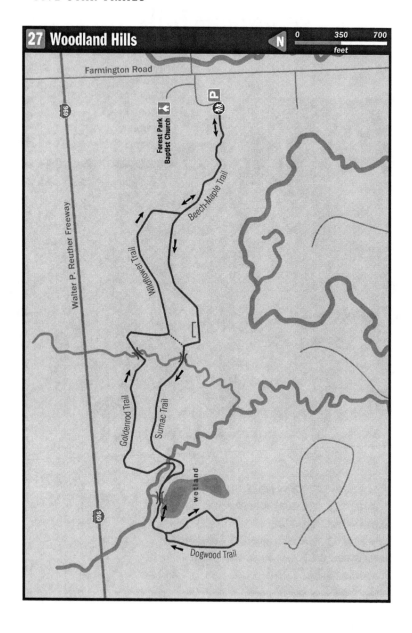

Overview

Woodland Hills is home to one of the last vestiges of beech-maple forests in southeastern Michigan. Never mind that the network of trails crisscrossing this nature park lies a stone's throw from busy I-696 in one of metro Detroit's busiest and most populous suburbs. Although the white noise of the highway is a constant reminder that civilization is not far away, you will find here a refuge from suburbia. The route meanders over gentle hills and through mature and young woods, tangled brush, and wetlands.

Route Details

Five trails combine to make up a 1.7-mile trek that snakes deep into the woods, with only an occasional glimpse of the highway. The flat Beech-Maple Trail begins on the western edge of the parking lot. The wide dirt path immediately crosses through thick foliage and patches of wildflowers, with the rumble of the interstate in the distance. Woodland Hills is a sanctuary for animals and their habitats; if you look closely, you'll likely see plenty of animal tracks. (The afternoon that I visited, I observed plenty of deer tracks along the trail, crossed paths with fluttering butterflies, and enjoyed the cacophony of chirping birds.)

At an intersection with the **Wildflower Trail,** continue straight along the **Beech-Maple Trail;** you'll hit the Wildflower Trail on the way back. As the trail stretches westward, the trees are taller and the sense of forest becomes more pronounced. Pass a pair of benches and descend a steep hill to a junction with the **Wildflower** and **Sumac** trails. Turn left on the **Sumac Trail,** easing downward to a long wooden bridge over a creek that ripples over scattered rocks and downed trees. (Looking up the stream, I noticed a beaver dam.)

The trail makes a steep climb beyond the creek before it levels and becomes a mowed, grassy path. The woods open up here. A grassy bank blanketed with purple flowers hides the interstate near the junction with the **Goldenrod Trail.** Veer left and follow the **Wildflower**

Trail south. The trail becomes dirt again, and the canopy of trees overhead creates the sensation of walking through a tunnel. Where the trail recrosses the creek, look for a small waterfall.

The trail comes to a T-junction at a fence marking private property. Turn right and follow the trail along the edge of a wetland, one of the highlights of this hike, along with the beech and maple trees. A bench provides a fine spot to take in the view. Reeds and cattails crowd the edge of the wetland. This pastoral landscape is interrupted only by a view of the interstate and vehicles screaming by. (On the afternoon I visited, I encountered no other hikers and enjoyed complete solitude. Ducks and geese swam along calm waters, and other birds were plentiful.)

A railed bridge crosses part of the wetland, affording views on either side. Daisies and other wildflowers dot the banks, which are thick with brush. The dirt trail turns into the **Dogwood Trail,** a loop at the far western edge of the park. The area is more densely wooded, and the trail is narrow in spots. A pair of blue spruce trees seems out of place in these woods of beeches and maples.

Continue clockwise around the **Dogwood Trail** until you close the loop. From here, retrace your route to the junction of the **Sumac** and **Goldenrod** trails. Here go straight (north) on the **Goldenrod Trail.**

The **Goldenrod Trail** is mostly grassy and is closest to the interstate, running nearly parallel to it for about 500 feet. Banks with purple flowers and white pines screen the view, but you can't ignore the vehicles zooming by. Eventually, however, the trail meanders back into heavy brush and trees, sloping deeper into the woods. After crossing a creek via an L-shaped wooden bridge, the trail levels.

Now the trail turns sharply right (south), away from the interstate. Just before the junction with the **Wildflower** and **Beech-Maple** trails, notice a huge oak tree on your right. At the junction, turn left on the **Wildflower Trail.** Scattered throughout this stretch of the forest are occasional majestic maple trees. The trail becomes a wide, grassy swath as it nears a T-junction with the **Beech-Maple Trail.** At the junction, turn left and retrace your route to the parking lot.

Nearby Activities

The William P. Holliday Forest and Wildlife Preserve stretches snakelike along the Middle Rouge River in western Wayne County. The 500-acre preserve, about 10 miles south along Farmington Road, is home to a virgin forest of beech, maple, and oak trees and a variety of wildlife, including white-tailed deer. The Nankin Mills Nature Center bookends the eastern end of the preserve. Three short trails traverse the park, while the Tonquish Trail runs 5.8 miles along the length of the preserve.

Directions

From Detroit, take I-75 north about 8 miles to I-696 west, Exit 61. Follow I-696 about 13 miles to Orchard Lake Road, Exit 5. Turn right and drive to 12 Mile Road. Turn left on 12 Mile Road and go about 1 mile to Farmington Road. Turn left. The entrance to Woodland Hills is on the right, about 0.4 miles.

From Ann Arbor, take US 23 north to M-14 east. Follow M-14 about 14 miles to I-275 north. Take I-275 about 6 miles to I-696 east. Follow to Orchard Lake Road, Exit 5. Turn left onto Orchard Lake Road and drive to 12 Mile Road. Turn left and go about 1 mile to Farmington Road. Turn left. The entrance to Woodland Hills is about 0.4 miles on the right.

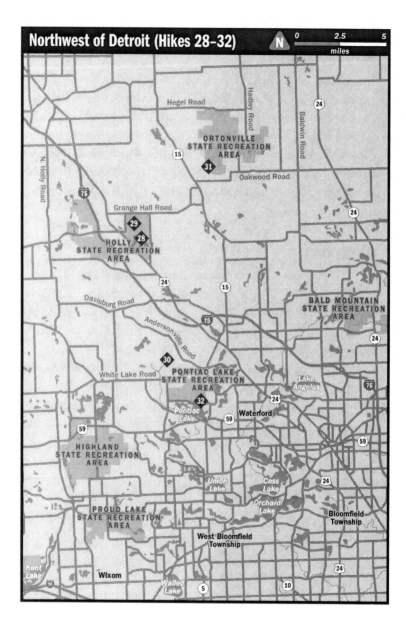

Northwest of Detroit (Hikes 28–32)

N

0   2.5   5
miles

Northwest of Detroit

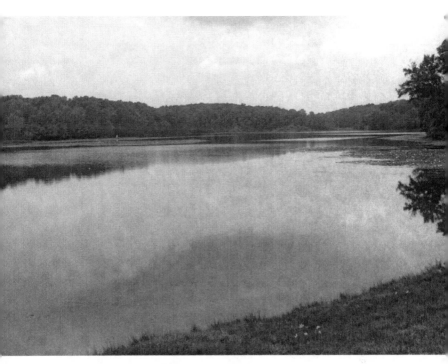

A VIEW OF MCGINNIS LAKE FROM A CLEARING

28 # Holly State Recreation Area: Lakeshore Trail

SCENERY: ★ ★ ★
TRAIL CONDITION: ★ ★ ★
CHILDREN: ★ ★ ★
DIFFICULTY: ★ ★
SOLITUDE: ★ ★ ★

A HILLTOP VIEW OF MCGINNIS LAKE

GPS TRAILHEAD COORDINATES: N42° 48.495' W83° 31.014'
DISTANCE & CONFIGURATION: 2.4-mile loop
HIKING TIME: About 1 hour
HIGHLIGHTS: Lakes, woodlands, wetlands
ELEVATION: 1,008 feet at trailhead; 1,097 feet at highest point
ACCESS: Daily, 8 a.m.–10 p.m.; $10 annual recreation passport per vehicle
MAPS: Available from the attendant at the tollbooth and **michigan.gov/org**
FACILITIES: Restrooms, picnic areas, campgrounds, volleyball, horseshoe pits
WHEELCHAIR ACCESS: None
COMMENTS: Trail is open to seasonal hunting.
CONTACTS: 248-634-8811; **michigan.gov/org**

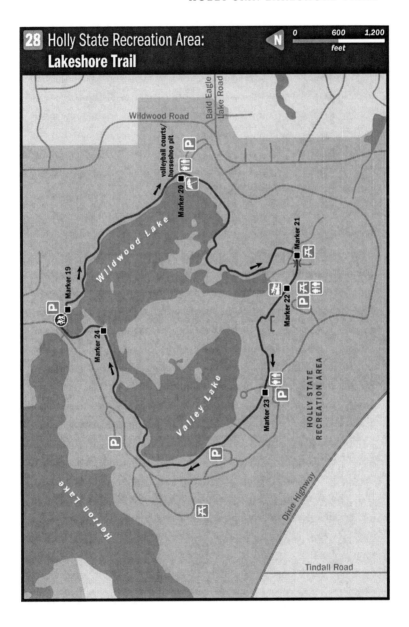

28 Holly State Recreation Area:
Lakeshore Trail

N

0   600   1,200
feet

Bald Eagle
Lake Road

Wildwood Road

volleyball courts/
horseshoe pit

Marker 20

Marker 21

Wildwood Lake

Marker 19

Marker 22

Marker 24

Valley Lake

Marker 23

HOLLY STATE
RECREATION AREA

Herron Lake

Dixie Highway

Tindall Road

Overview

At the Holly State Recreation Area, you'll find dense woodlands, open fields, wetlands, quiet streams, and several lakes, most of them filled with anglers in the warm months. Long stretches of the Lakeshore Trail wrap around Wildwood Lake and Valley Lake, with ample views of these serene waters. Occasionally, the trail veers away from the water and deeper into the woods. Although the hiking is easy, the route has a few hills, and the short climb to the crest of one offers a panoramic view of Valley Lake.

Route Details

With just 7,800 acres, the Holly State Recreation Area in northern Oakland County may pale in comparison to many of Michigan's larger state parks and recreation areas, but its gently rolling hills offer varied scenery and 10 miles of hiking trails. Ten natural lakes dot the landscape, and they attract anglers, boaters, and swimmers. The park also offers sheltered and open picnic areas, campgrounds, and rustic cabins, making it one of the busiest weekend retreats in southeastern Michigan, drawing about 350,000 visitors a year. Like other state recreation areas, portions of the trail are open to seasonal hunting. My advice is to avoid the trail during firearms season, which is mid- to late November.

Despite its proximity to the sprawling Detroit suburbs, much of the Holly State Recreation Area was created from undeveloped land. That's because most of the park has been in the hands of the state for decades, long before development began spreading northward from Detroit. Michigan bought a good share of the tract—3,466 acres—in 1943 but didn't designate the land as a recreation area until five years later. In the early 1950s, the recreation area nearly doubled in size, to 6,017 acres, and included skiing facilities. But the state eventually sold the ski area to a private developer. From the park's entrance, you can still see the ski lifts from the Mt. Holly ski area.

Many improvements to the park have been made over the years—cabins, shelters, picnic tables, restrooms, and boat ramps—but much of the land remains free from human intrusions. One of the few remnants of the past is a rustic cabin built in 1938. The cabin was once the staging area for turkey shoots and a gathering place for friends. Secluded among old-growth hardwoods, spruce trees, and a small reflecting pond, the cabin is hardly noticeable near the park entrance.

To reach the Lakeshore trailhead, about 70 feet from the parking lot, head down a grassy slope. You will pass a picnic area that affords a panoramic view of Wildwood Lake and anglers casting their lines along the shore. The Lakeshore Trail lives up to its name, following the shoreline of Wildwood Lake as the path cuts into thick brush and woods. The trail parallels the shoreline for a long stretch, giving hikers the sense that they are practically walking on water and offering an unobstructed view of the serene lake. Downed trees litter the shoreline, with occasional splashes of wildflowers along the banks. Above the trail, the terrain is thick with vegetation and new-growth trees.

The landscape here is typical of southeastern Michigan: a mix of natural lakes, swamps, open fields, woods, and gently rolling hills. The Holly State Recreation Area has five trails, but the Lakeshore Trail is the only one that runs along the perimeters of two lakes—Wildwood Lake and Valley Lake. Wildlife is abundant: look for Canada geese, white-tailed deer, rabbits, and squirrels. Occasionally you'll hear the scattering of a ruffed grouse in the brush or happen across a pheasant in an open field. Stretches of the trail cross swampy areas, so don't be surprised to see a snake slither across your route. Within 0.3 miles, you'll reach marker 19 at a fork in the trail. Be sure to continue southeast along the edge of the lake to marker 20. The other path at that fork leads to a picnic and parking area.

As you approach marker 20, the trail exits the woods and opens up to a well-used picnic area, complete with restrooms, picnic tables, a grill, a small sandy volleyball court, and a horseshoe pit. Expect to find a family or two picnicking here during the warmer months. To continue, follow the mowed swath of grass back into the woodlands and cross a cattail-fringed marsh, meandering along the southern shoreline of Wildwood Lake.

Around the 1-mile mark, the trail veers away from the lake and the terrain becomes slightly hilly and thick with woods. The stretch between Wildwood Lake and Valley Lake is swampy, with reeds and cattails lining the trail. Lily pads and wildflowers are plentiful along the shore. At marker 21, the trail crosses a small wooden bridge over a creek and then rises above the lake through the woods. You'll find a pavilion and picnic area on your left, just before the trail again steers away from the shoreline, rising above another swampy area.

After you cross another small wooden bridge, the terrain becomes hillier. At marker 22, the trail crosses a driveway leading to a boat ramp. A parking area is at your left. The trail gradually slopes to a creek and a swamp before eventually rising again. At the crest of the hill, you are rewarded with a panoramic view of Valley Lake. Near the 1.8-mile mark, two benches invite a moment's rest. The benches are well anchored, so there are no worries about falling backward into the sloping brush. A split-rail fence prevents anyone from falling forward over a short cliff. Just beyond this rest spot are a picnic table, a grill, and a parking lot.

From here, the trail passes among towering maple trees and rises above the lake. The trail wraps around Valley Lake, and eases down to the shoreline. Once again, you'll see anglers casting their lines and boats drifting on the water. The trail runs along the northern end of the lake, just below a paved park road, before closing the loop near the picnic area. From here, retrace your route to the parking lot.

Nearby Activities

About 5 miles northeast, the Ortonville State Recreation Area is about half the size of the Holly State Recreation Area, with 5,400 acres, and offers similar outdoor activities, including hiking, biking, swimming, and boating. The 2.5-mile Ortonville Hiking–Mountain Bike Trail is well used by cyclists and hikers. The Mt. Holly ski area is about 6 miles east of the park, just off I-75 or Dixie Highway.

Directions

From Detroit, take I-75 north to Exit 101 (Grange Hall Road). Turn right on Grange Hall Road and go about 1 mile to McGinnis Road. Veer right and continue about 0.8 miles to the park entrance. The parking lot for the Lakeshore Trailhead is about 0.8 miles beyond the attendant's gate.

From Ann Arbor, take US 23 north to Silver Lake Road, Exit 23. Turn right and head west on Silver Lake Road. It eventually becomes Main Street and then turns into Grange Hall Road. Follow Grange Hall Road about 8 miles to McGinnis Road. Veer right and continue about 0.8 miles to the park entrance. The parking lot for the Lakeshore Trailhead is about 0.8 miles past the attendant's gate.

29 Holly State Recreation Area: Wilderness Trail

SCENERY: ★ ★ ★
TRAIL CONDITION: ★ ★ ★
CHILDREN: ★ ★ ★
DIFFICULTY: ★ ★
SOLITUDE: ★ ★ ★

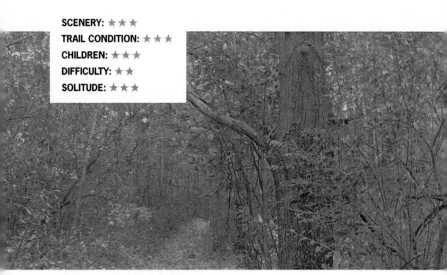

STATELY TREES DOT THE LANDSCAPE.

GPS TRAILHEAD COORDINATES: N42° 49.269' W83° 31.679'
DISTANCE & CONFIGURATION: 4.7-mile loop
HIKING TIME: About 2 hours
HIGHLIGHTS: Woodlands, wetlands, McGinnis Lake
ELEVATION: 1,022 at trailhead, with no significant rise
ACCESS: Daily, 8 a.m.–10 p.m.; $10 annual recreation passport per vehicle
MAPS: Available from the attendant at the tollbooth and **michigan.gov/org**
FACILITIES: Restrooms, picnic areas, campgrounds
WHEELCHAIR ACCESS: None
COMMENTS: The trail passes through some areas open to seasonal hunting.
CONTACTS: 248-634-8811; **michigan.gov/dnr**

Overview

The Wilderness Trail traverses some of the most rolling and wooded terrain in the Holly State Recreation Area and northern Oakland

County. The trail remains primarily in the woods, thick with oaks, maples, and beeches, and passes ponds and wetlands as it circles around McGinnis Lake.

Route Details

The Wilderness Trail is the longest of the hiking trails at Holly State Recreation Area and is located north of McGinnis Road in a more secluded area of the park. More than 30 miles of trails are located in the Holly State Recreation Area, and all of them are open to hikers. However, the Holdridge Mountain Bike Trail in the western section of the park, on the opposite side of I-75, is dominated by bikers. Most hikers steer to the Lakeshore and Wilderness trails. The latter also is open to bikers.

For hikers, the best bets are this Wilderness Trail and the Lakeshore Trail (see page 172), found in the eastern section of the park and straddling McGinnis Road. The Wilderness Trail is the longer of the two. The trails, however, are connected and can be combined for a nearly 8-mile hike. There is no name for the trail connecting the two; the state's marker system starts at the trailhead of the Wilderness Trail and continues in sequence to marker 15. To connect to the Lakeshore Trail, hikers can head south from markers 11 or 12 to markers 16, 17, 18, and 19. Marker 19 is the trailhead for the Lakeshore Trail.

For the most part, the Wilderness Trail winds through woodlands as it makes its way around McGinnis Lake. There are few man-made intrusions, other than a dirt road and a campground on the south side of the lake.

You may pick up the Wilderness Trail in several places. The park identifies the main trailhead south of McGinnis Road at the Overlook Picnic Area. Signage marks a second parking lot as Wilderness Trailhead. Marker 17 notes the trail. You also may access the trail off McGinnis Road as well as Wildwood Road.

For this hike, I began at marker 1. This trailhead is located just off the park road, beyond the small parking area and the attendant's

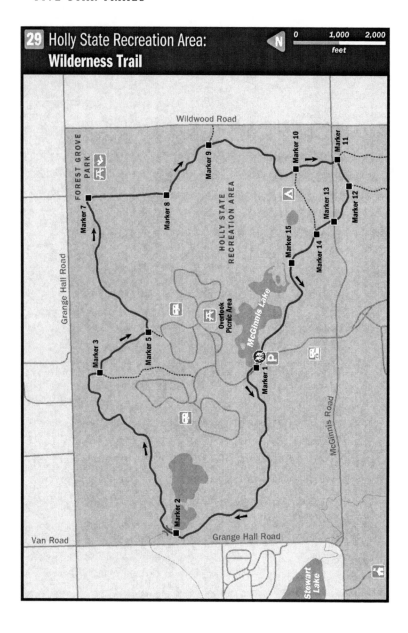

booth. Walk across the causeway that crosses a narrow stretch of a small lake. You'll see marker 1 on the left (west) of the road in the brush. The trail slopes gently into thin woods and narrows as it heads west to marker 2.

The trail winds through gently rolling woodlands, with occasional ponds and wetlands. Pines also are prominent in the forest here. Near the 0.5-mile mark, the trail crosses a meadow, and Stewart Lake is visible on the southern horizon. Marker 2 stands near a small marshy pond at the 0.9-mile mark.

From here, the trail veers north-northeast, crosses a small bridge, and runs deeper into the hardwood forest. Marker 3 is at the 1.6-mile mark. Continue straight at this intersection to marker 5. If you had headed south to marker 4, you would reach a campground at McGinnis Lake, where there are public restrooms.

This stretch of the trail is hilly and dotted with wetlands. The trail drops about 60 feet before reaching a marshy pond and then rises briefly to marker 5. Another spur leads to a campground; continue northeast to marker 7. Around the 2-mile mark, the trail emerges from tree cover and the sides become thick with brush. This is a particularly hilly stretch, with the trail rising and dipping.

Marker 7 is posted near the 2.5-mile mark near Forest Grove Park, which has a playground and picnic area. Swing right, heading south into the woods. The landscape changes little, with the trail winding through hilly woodlands and past marshes to markers 8 and 9. Marker 9 is posted at the 3-mile mark.

The trail then runs along the crest of a hill with a steep embankment on your right and an expansive wetland below. At an unmarked T-intersection, turn left and continue straight (avoid any spurs). This leads to marker 10 at the edge of a campground. Continue straight through the campground and across McGinnis Road to marker 11.

From there, head west; markers 12, 13, 14, and 15 are within 0.5 miles. From marker 15, the trail rises and affords impressive views of marshy stretches of McGinnis Lake. Continue heading west along the lake for your return to marker 1 to complete the hike.

Nearby Attractions

About 14 miles southwest, the Drayton Plains Nature Center offers a series of trails that loop around the former ponds of a state fish hatchery, no longer in use. The landscape is largely open, but some of the trails run along the Clinton River and thin woodlands. The 137-acre tract attracts plenty of birds and waterfowl and a host of mammals often can be seen roaming the grounds. The interpretive center, formerly the living quarters of the men who worked the ponds, serves as administrative offices and houses native mammals, reptiles, and birds in re-created habitat, as well as a gift shop.

Directions

From Detroit, take I-75 north to Exit 101 (Grange Hall Road). Turn right on Grange Hall Road and go about 1 mile to McGinnis Road. Veer right and continue about 0.8 miles to the park entrance.

From Ann Arbor, take US 23 north to Silver Lake Road, Exit 23. Turn right and head west on Silver Lake Road. It eventually becomes Main Street and then turns into Grange Hall Road. Follow Grange Hall Road about 8 miles to McGinnis Road. Veer right and continue about 0.8 miles to the park entrance.

30

Indian Springs Metropark: Woodland and Timberland Lake Trails

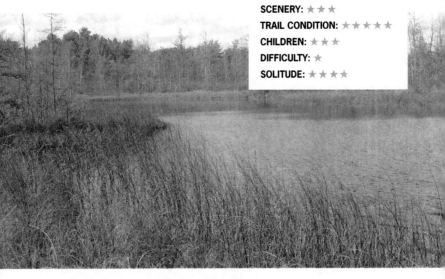

SCENERY: ★ ★ ★
TRAIL CONDITION: ★ ★ ★ ★
CHILDREN: ★ ★ ★
DIFFICULTY: ★
SOLITUDE: ★ ★ ★

TIMBERLAND LAKE IS A REWARD FOR HIKERS.

GPS TRAILHEAD COORDINATES: N42° 70.778' W83° 48.789'

DISTANCE & CONFIGURATION: 3.6-mile loop and spur

HIKING TIME: About 1 hour

HIGHLIGHTS: Woodlands, marshes, boardwalks, Timberland Lake

ELEVATION: 996 feet at trailhead, with no significant rise

ACCESS: April–October, 7 a.m.–10 p.m.; November–March, 7 a.m.–8 p.m.; $5 per day or $25 per year

MAPS: Available at the park visitor center or **metroparks.com**

FACILITIES: Visitor center, restrooms, picnic areas, golf course, playground

WHEELCHAIR ACCESS: Yes

COMMENTS: No biking, jogging, or pets are allowed on the trail. Beware of the eastern massasauga rattlesnake, which inhabits the area.

CONTACTS: 248-625-6640; **metroparks.com**

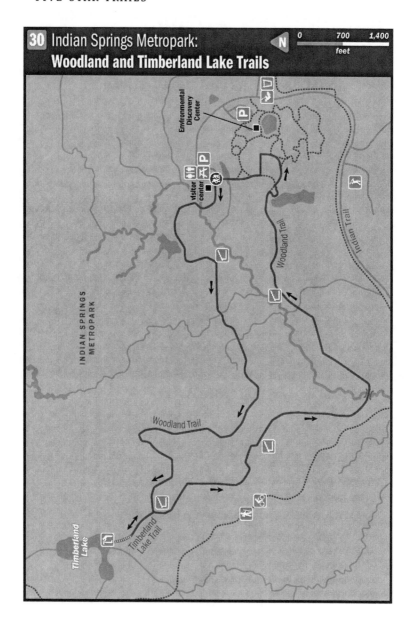

30 Indian Springs Metropark:
Woodland and Timberland Lake Trails

Overview

The longest of the nature trails at Indian Springs Metropark, the Woodland Trail runs deep into wet forests and through fields and meadows en route to secluded Timberland Lake. A long boardwalk leads to the lake, cutting through a marsh thick with cattails and reeds. This trail is particularly beautiful in the spring, when wildflowers are in bloom, and in the fall, when the towering oaks and maples are ablaze with brilliant autumn colors.

Route Details

At just 2,215 acres, Indian Springs Metropark is one of the smallest of southeast Detroit's Metropark System. But the area, known as the Huron Swamp, had the distinction of being the largest undeveloped natural area in southeast Michigan when the Huron-Clinton Metropolitan Authority began acquiring land for the park in 1974.

Located 9 miles northwest of the city of Pontiac and at the headwaters of the Huron River, Indian Springs offers 6 miles of self-guided nature trails that meander through wet woodlands, meadows, and fields outside the park's nature center. A series of smaller hikes leads from outside the Environmental Discovery Center. They loop around ponds, a marsh, a native plant garden, and short-grass and tallgrass prairies.

The Woodland Trail offers a beautiful hike deep in the woods, dominated by towering oaks, maples, and beech trees. The trail begins at the end of the pavement right outside the nature center. A wide grassy swath leads into the woods, where you will see warning signs for the eastern massasauga rattlesnake: this stretch is prime habitat for this reptile.

As you walk along the wide dirt trail, you'll notice freshly cut trees, the victims of emerald ash borer beetles. The first in a series of boardwalks crosses through a tamarack swamp; tamaracks, if you don't know, are the only conifers to lose their needles in the fall. They stand out in the fall as their needles turn a brownish-orange. The first of four intersections (they're simply loop shortcuts) en route to Timberland Lake comes at around 0.3 miles. Bear right at each one of them. At the first one, you'll see a sign that notes the 3.5-mile hike to and from Timberland Lake. The lake is located at about the halfway point of this hike.

The trail crosses yet another boardwalk through a marsh, thick with brush, reeds, and ferns. You'll hear plenty of warblers and other birds, and you might want to bring your binoculars to catch sight of pileated woodpeckers, great horned owls, or red-shouldered hawks.

Small posts label noteworthy trees, including sugar maple, shagbark hickory, basswood, beech, wild black cherry, white oak, and tulip tree. There's also a vegetation enclosure study plot, a small fenced-in area that is being studied to gauge the impact that white-tailed deer have had on the surrounding landscape.

The Woodland Trail winds deeper into the woods and more wetlands, dotted with downed and uprooted trees and rich with ferns and tamaracks. Another long boardwalk leads to the 0.1-mile-long Timberland Lake Trail, which cuts through a sedge fen bordering the lake. Despite the seclusion of this site, don't be surprised to hear the rumbling of cars and trucks in the distance.

From the Timberland Lake Trail, veer right and continue southeastward as the trail loops back toward the nature center. Along the trail you'll spot the rusted remains of an old woodstove someone found in the swamp. A sign speculates about its past, whether it was part of an old logging camp, small cabin, or hunting lodge. A rain shelter is nearby; stay to the right as the trail intersects with shortcuts from the northern stretch of the trail.

The trail turns into a grassy swath as it leaves the woods, thick with brush; smaller, thinner trees; wildflowers; and trembling aspens. As you approach the nature center, you'll see the park's golf course and hills dotted with trees in the distance. Continue just a short distance and you'll intersect with pathways leading back to the nature center. A native plant garden nearby identifies flowers and fauna from the nearby woods.

Nearby Attractions

Just down the road, about 9 miles southeast, is the Pontiac Lake State Recreation Area, which offers outdoor enthusiasts a wealth of activities, including hiking, mountain biking, fishing, swimming, and boating. The 3,745-acre park also draws equestrians, cross-country skiers, and hunters. The 3,800-acre park boasts three campgrounds and is home to an equestrian staging area and day-use facilities. The latter include a concession stand, beach, and bathhouse at Pontiac Lake. The 11-mile Pontiac Lake Mountain Bike Trail is a favorite of hikers and trail runners.

Directions

From Detroit, take I-75 north to Dixie Highway, Exit 93. Turn left onto Dixie Highway (US 24) and drive about 1.7 miles to White Lake Road. Turn right and go about 1.7 miles to Andersonville Road. Turn right and go about 0.5 miles to White Lake Road. Turn left and go 3.3 miles to Indian Trail. Turn right. The park is on your right.

From Ann Arbor, take US 23 north to M-59, Exit 67. Turn right and head east toward Pontiac and drive about 10 miles, passing Ormand Road. Then make a Michigan U-turn (to reach the opposite side of the road, you have to turn left into the median and then continue) to head west on M-59. Go 0.2 miles and turn right onto Ormond Road. Drive 2.6 miles and turn right onto White Lake Road. Go 2.2 miles and turn left onto Indian Trail. The park is on the right.

31

Ortonville State Recreation Area:

Hiking—Mountain Bike Trail

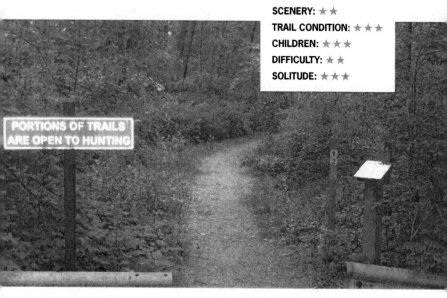

SCENERY: ★ ★
TRAIL CONDITION: ★ ★ ★
CHILDREN: ★ ★ ★
DIFFICULTY: ★ ★
SOLITUDE: ★ ★ ★

PORTIONS OF TRAILS
ARE OPEN TO HUNTING

MANY STATE-PARK TRAILS PASS THROUGH SEASONAL HUNTING AREAS.

GPS TRAILHEAD COORDINATES: N42° 52.124' W83° 26.300'

DISTANCE & CONFIGURATION: 2.5-mile loop

HIKING TIME: About 1 hour

HIGHLIGHTS: Woodlands, fields

ELEVATION: 1,042 feet at trailhead, with no significant rise

ACCESS: Daily, 8 a.m.–10 p.m.; $10 annual recreation passport per vehicle

MAPS: At **michigan.gov/dnr**

FACILITIES: None

WHEELCHAIR ACCESS: None

COMMENTS: Portions of the trail are open to hunting. Pets must be kept on a 6-foot leash.

CONTACTS: 810-797-4439; **michigan.gov/org**

Overview

Located in a more secluded area and in the oldest section of the Ortonville State Recreation Area, this easy-to-follow trail loops through a densely wooded forest and occasional fields. Some stretches of the trail are hilly but never overly strenuous.

Route Details

The 5,400-acre state recreation area straddling northern Oakland and southern Lapeer counties offers a little bit of everything for outdoor enthusiasts amid its hilly, wooded terrain: here you have trails for hiking, mountain biking, horseback riding, snowmobiling, and cross-country skiing.

Hikers and mountain bikers share a 2.5-mile trail in the area known as Bloomer #3 State Park in the southwestern corner of the recreation area. This area was the original park and is named after the man who donated the land to the state in 1922. Development of the area for recreation began in earnest in 1945, and land acquisitions over the years have expanded the park to its current size. Tucked away on a wooded hillside in this area is a single rustic pine cabin. It's available for rentals and includes propane heat, a vault toilet, and a grill.

The trailhead is about 100 feet off State Park Road. The trail begins just to the right of a large wooden park information sign and a self-registration table (at this location, the state uses the honor system to collect daily-use fees). The trail is well marked, using the standard state park sign system with numbered posts. In addition, posts with arrows noting trail direction are scattered along the trail.

From marker 1, the trail slips immediately into the woods. Both sides of the trail are thick with brush, and you'll notice pine trees here and there. The trail winds through dense woods and brush and gradually rises. The trail dips throughout much of the loop, but it's never strenuous. For the most part, the landscape changes very

189

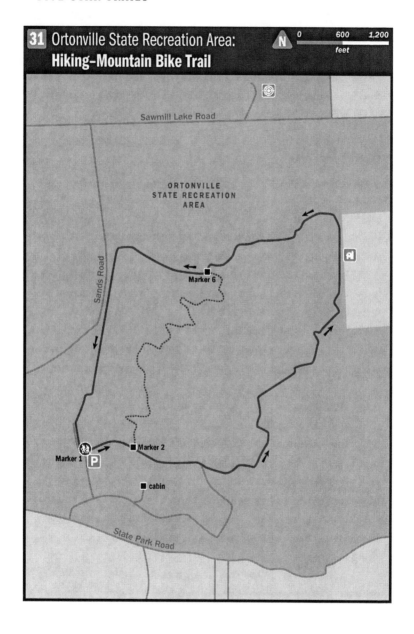

31 Ortonville State Recreation Area:
Hiking–Mountain Bike Trail

N

0   600   1,200
feet

ORTONVILLE
STATE RECREATION
AREA

Sawmill Lake Road

Sands Road

Marker 6

Marker 2

Marker 1

P

cabin

State Park Road

little. Although several small lakes dot the park, none of them come close to the trail. Hikers are mostly trekking through dense woods, broken only occasionally by fields.

Marker 2 stands near the 0.1-mile point. At this juncture, hikers can follow a shortcut to marker 6, which stretches due north and dissects the loop in half. A sign here also points out a cross-country ski trail. To continue around the loop, stay east. The dirt trail narrows but is framed by wide grassy shoulders.

Marker 3 is about 0.2 miles northeast. The trail follows the crest of a hill, with steep slopes on either side, thick with hardwood trees and shrubs. Even though you're deep in the woods, don't be surprised to hear the muffled sounds of traffic nearby. Heading toward marker 4, the trail dips in several spots, with wildflowers scattered along both sides of the trail.

At about the 0.6-mile mark, swing right; keep an eye out for a signpost with an arrow. Marker 4 stands near the 0.8-mile mark. Expect to hear the echo of gunshots along this stretch; the park's shooting range is located just north of the trail, off Sawmill Lake Road. The first break in the woods, a small field, comes into view after marker 4, but the trail retreats back into the woods within 0.1 mile.

The tree line begins to thin on the right around the 1-mile mark. The cultivated fields of the neighboring farm are barely visible through the trees and brush in the warm months. Hikers will catch a glimpse of a barn just as the trail ducks under a thicker canopy of trees.

Look for marker 5 around the 1.3-mile mark. Continue west to marker 6, another 0.4 miles ahead. At marker 6, hikers can opt for a more direct path back to the starting point: just swing left or south. To continue along the longer loop, veer right to marker 7. Wildflowers and wild berries grow in scattered patches along the trail. Wild turkeys are plentiful along this stretch; try not to startle a hen and her brood.

Marker 7 stands near the 2-mile mark in a small clearing. Follow the trail left into the woods. The grassy trail edges along the bottom of a hill and the woods become thinner. At about the 2.3-mile mark, pine trees stand sentinel along the trail. Just up ahead, the trail bends and a wooden sign with arrows points the way back to the trailhead.

Nearby Attractions

A number of state and county parks surround Ortonville State Recreation Area, including Metamora State Recreation Area, Holly State Recreation Area, Seven Lakes State Park, and Grove Land Oaks and Independence Oaks county parks (the latter two are Oakland County parks). All of these parks are home to networks of hiking trails. About 15 miles southwest of the Ortonville State Recreation Area, the 1,400-acre Seven Lakes State Park, its name calling your attention to the seven lakes that dot the park, opened in 1992 and is one of Michigan's newest state parks. At Seven Lakes, you can enjoy several short hiking trails, including the longest one, the 2.1-mile Green Trail Loop.

Directions

From Detroit, take I-75 north to Exit 91, M-15 (Ortonville Road). Drive about 8 miles and turn right on Oakwood Road. Go about 0.9 miles and then turn left on Sands Road. Continue about 0.5 miles and turn right on State Park Road. The entrance to the trailhead is about 0.3 miles on your left.

From Ann Arbor, take US 23 north to Silver Lake Road, Exit 79. Turn right and follow West Silver Lake Road for about 1.3 miles. West Silver Lake Road turns into Main Street and then becomes Grange Hall Road after about 8 miles. Continue for another 5 miles along Grange Hall Road to M-15. Turn left onto M-15 (Ortonville

Road). Turn left on M-15 and follow it about 0.5 miles to Oakwood Road. Turn right on Oakwood Road and go about 0.9 miles to Sands Road. Turn left on Sands Road. Go about 0.5 miles and then turn right onto State Park Road. The park entrance is about 0.3 miles on your left.

32

Pontiac Lake State Recreation Area:
Campground to Beach Trail

SCENERY: ★ ★ ★
TRAIL CONDITION: ★ ★ ★ ★
CHILDREN: ★ ★ ★
DIFFICULTY: ★ ★
SOLITUDE: ★ ★ ★

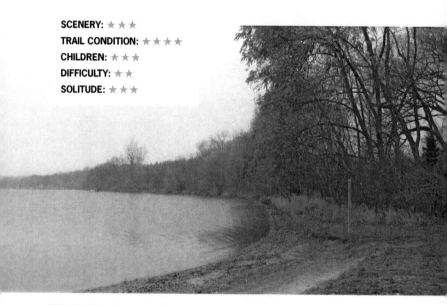

THE BEACH AREA AT PONTIAC LAKE

GPS TRAILHEAD COORDINATES: N42° 40.290' W83° 26.967'

DISTANCE & CONFIGURATION: 4-mile out-and-back

HIKING TIME: About 2 hours

HIGHLIGHTS: Woodlands, marshes, fields, Pontiac Lake

ELEVATION: 966 feet at trailhead, with gradual 100-foot rises; 1,130 feet at highest point

ACCESS: Daily, 8 a.m.–10 p.m.; $10 annual recreation passport per vehicle

MAPS: At **michigan.gov/dnr**

FACILITIES: Restrooms, picnic areas, playground, concession store, beach, campgrounds

WHEELCHAIR ACCESS: None

COMMENTS: The trail intersects and converges with the Equestrian Trail at several points. Bicycles are prohibited. Hunting is allowed in some areas of the park in season.

CONTACTS: 248-666-1020; **michigan.gov/dnr**

Overview

The only hiking trail—which is labeled Campground to Beach on the official map—begins just off the beach at Pontiac Lake. It passes through heavy woods, marshlands, and old farm fields to the park's modern campground. Some of the terrain is rolling, making for moderately strenuous hiking on occasion. Not to be missed is the trail's scenic vista with sweeping views of the countryside south of the park.

Route Details

Just off busy M-59, the Pontiac Lake State Recreation Area is an oasis among the sprawl stretching west from Pontiac, the Oakland County seat. The focal point is 585-acre Pontiac Lake, created in 1926 when Lime Lake, a smaller lake in the upper Huron River watershed, was dammed.

Several islands and peninsulas dot Pontiac Lake, but unfortunately, the Campground to Beach Trail runs nowhere near them. Except for a panoramic view from a short spur, the lake remains largely invisible to hikers; you will hear, however, the roar of speedboats and motorboats during the summer. Among outdoor enthusiasts, the hiking trail is overshadowed by the popular 11-mile Mountain Bike Trail and the 17-mile Equestrian Trail. Hiking is permitted on the Mountain Bike Trail, but take note: the trail is heavily used by mountain bikers and trail runners.

The Campground to Beach Trail cuts through the center of the 3,745-acre park and intersects with the Equestrian and Mountain Bike trails. Even so, hikers will find long stretches of solitude once the trail passes park roads and continues northwesterly toward the campgrounds.

The trailhead for the hiking trail is a bit difficult to find. You'll immediately see the trailhead for both the Mountain Bike and Equestrian trails at the northwest corner of the parking lot off Gale Road. The trailhead for the Campground to Beach Trail begins at the

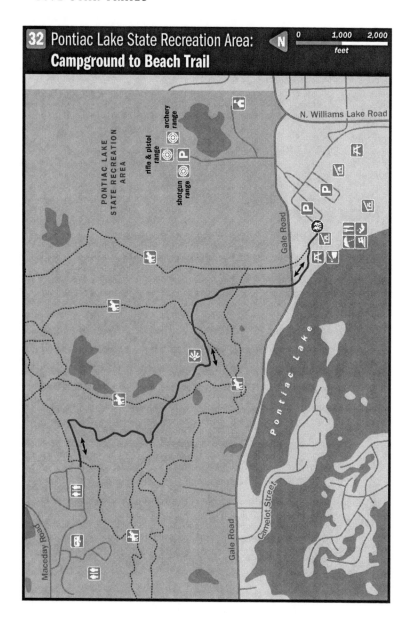

32 Pontiac Lake State Recreation Area:
Campground to Beach Trail

N

0   1,000   2,000
feet

N. Williams Lake Road

PONTIAC LAKE
STATE RECREATION
AREA

archery range

rifle & pistol range

shotgun range

Gale Road

Pontiac Lake

Camelot Street

Gale Road

Maceday Road

northern edge of the picnic area beyond the beach, about 1,000 feet northwest of the parking lot. A wooden sign simply notes the hiking path and the 1.8-mile distance to the campgrounds.

While the hiking trail circumvents the main geographic feature of the park, Pontiac Lake, it manages to pass through the other notable landscapes, including marshes, ponds, rolling woodlands, and old farm fields. The trail quickly departs the beach and the hustle and bustle of the park just as soon as you pass through old farm fields and cross Gale Road, about 500 feet from the trailhead.

The spur to the grassy knoll, which offers a panoramic view of the region, comes around the 0.1-mile mark. The spur is marked as an Equestrian Trail, but if the path is clear of horseback riders, walk about 0.2 miles to a clearing on your left; the spur continues far beyond that, but you can pause here for the view and then return to the main trail. From this vantage point, the only man-made structures in sight are the control tower, hangars, and other buildings of nearby Oakland County International Airport to the east. Otherwise, you can see tree canopy stretching for miles.

Turn around and head back to the main trail. The trail widens as it approaches a pair of majestic oak trees on your right, just before a junction with the Mountain Bike Trail at the 0.7-mile mark.

The woods become thicker, and the trail winds around marshes and ponds as it continues northwest to the campground. In early

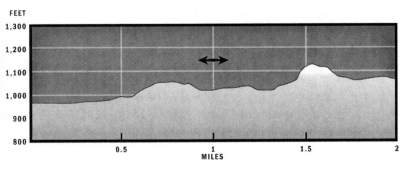

spring, many of the low-lying woodlands are flooded, and at those times you can expect muddy, wet stretches along the trail.

From about the 0.9-mile point, the terrain becomes hilly and passes through ravines. Except for occasional intersections with the Equestrian and Mountain Bike trails, the landscape from this point to the campground remains largely the same: woodlands thick with black and white oak and beech trees.

Still, there are some things to watch out for on this part of the trail, such as deep ravines, gently flowing streams, and beautiful swaths of forest. At that 0.9-mile mark, swing left at the intersection of trails. For the most part, the trail is well marked, with yellow signposts identifying the footpath. Near the 1.2-mile mark, turn right down a hill and along a rocky path. Occasionally, white pines break up the monotony of the hardwoods. Around the 1.4-mile mark, the trail reaches a T-intersection. Turn right, passing a pond and wetlands. The path separates from its convergence with the Equestrian Trail and continues around the swamp.

The trail eventually rises and follows the crest of a hill before descending past a stand of white pines and on to the campground. No signs mark the approach to the campground, though you might hear campers in busy season. But at the 2.2-mile mark, swing left at the T-intersection and take an immediate right. The trail abruptly ends at the campgrounds. There's nothing noteworthy to see here. Turn around and retrace your steps to the beach.

Nearby Activities

If you're looking for other recreational activities, the park also offers fishing, wintertime cross-country skiing and snowmobiling, hunting, and a shooting range. The lake is accessible by boat: a public ramp is located at the east end of the lake, with boat rentals and a marina at the western end. Shore fishing is allowed along the 0.3-mile-long beach and from a fishing pier. A concession stand, picnic areas, ball fields, and a playground are among the amenities for day visitors.

The park also is home to three campgrounds. While the 3,745-acre park boasts a wealth of recreational activities, hikers will find only one other trail designated specifically for their enjoyment. The 11-mile Mountain Bike Trail is open to hikers but is predominantly used by trail runners and bikers. If you're looking for solitude, you won't find it on this trail.

The Highland State Recreation Area, about 10 miles to the west on M-59, caters largely to mountain-bike riders and equestrians, but the 5,900-acre park also boasts a few hiking trails. They are centered on the remains of the former Edsel Ford cottage and some are shared with horseback riders. Most of the hiking and equestrian trails begin near a barn and other structures, part of the former estate of Edsel and Eleanor Ford. The Green Trail passes through the Haven Hill Natural Area, home to all of Michigan's principal forest types within one small area. They include a swamp forest of tamarack and cedar, a beech-maple forest, an oak-hickory forest, and a mixed hardwood forest. The area has remained largely undisturbed for the past 75 years.

Directions

From Detroit, take I-75 north to Exit 77, M-59, about 30 miles from downtown Detroit. Follow M-59 west about 8 miles. Turn right on North Williams Lake Road. The park entrance is about 1 mile north on the left-hand side.

From Ann Arbor, on M-14 and US 23, follow US 23 north about 23 miles to Exit 67, M-59. Continue east on M-59 about 17 miles to North Williams Lake Road. Turn left. The park entrance is about 1 mile north on the left-hand side.

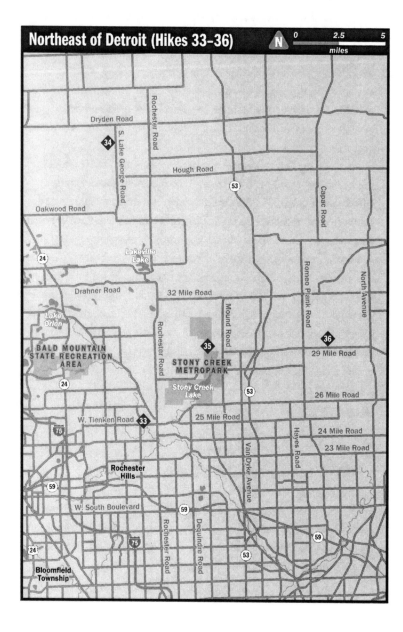

Northeast of Detroit

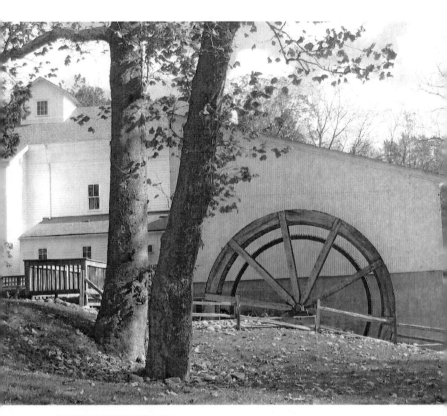

THE HISTORIC WOLCOTT MILL

Paint Creek Trail

SCENERY: ★ ★ ★
TRAIL CONDITION: ★ ★ ★ ★ ★
CHILDREN: ★ ★ ★ ★ ★
DIFFICULTY: ★
SOLITUDE: ★

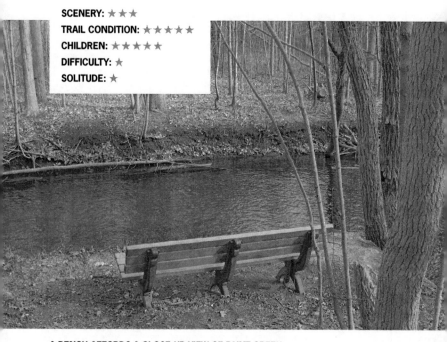

A BENCH AFFORDS A CLOSE-UP VIEW OF PAINT CREEK.

GPS TRAILHEAD COORDINATES: N42° 41.740' W83° 8.889'

DISTANCE & CONFIGURATION: 4.4-mile out-and-back

HIKING TIME: About 1.5 hours

HIGHLIGHTS: Woodlands, prairie, marshlands, Paint Creek

ELEVATION: 784 feet at trailhead; 830 feet at highest point

ACCESS: Daily, 6 a.m.–10 p.m.; no fees or permits required

MAPS: At the brochure boxes at various points along the trail, including the trailhead off West Tienken Road, and **paintcreektrail.org**

FACILITIES: Picnic area

WHEELCHAIR ACCESS: Yes

COMMENTS: Dogs are allowed on leashes. Horseback riding is allowed along some stretches.

CONTACTS: 248-651-9260; **paintcreektrail.org**

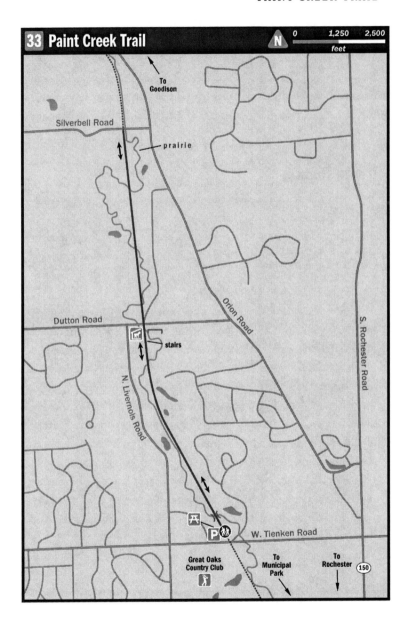

33 Paint Creek Trail

N

0   1,250   2,500
feet

To Goodison

Silverbell Road

prairie

Orion Road

Dutton Road

stairs

N. Livernois Road

S. Rochester Road

W. Tienken Road

P

Great Oaks Country Club

To Municipal Park

To Rochester   150

Overview

The stretch of the Paint Creek Trail from Tienken Road to Silverbell Road is among the most scenic of the 8.9-mile linear park. The trail passes under beautiful canopies of trees as it runs parallel to Paint Creek, crosses three bridges, and skirts marshlands and the remnant of a prairie.

Route Details

The Paint Creek Trail boasts the distinction of being the first rail-trail in Michigan and today is also one of the busiest in southeast Michigan, drawing more than 100,000 people a year. They come to walk, run, bike, ride horses, and, in the winter, cross-country ski on the wide, crushed-limestone surface trail. The trail was designated as a National Recreation Trail in 2006.

Stretching through picturesque northeast Oakland County, from Rochester to Lake Orion, the rail-trail was created from the former right-of-way of the Penn Central Railroad and opened to the public in 1983. The trail follows the meandering Paint Creek, which flows southeasterly into the Clinton River and is one of two designated trout streams in Oakland County. The thin woods along the trail are home to myriad wildlife, including white-tailed deer, foxes, squirrels, rabbits, raccoons, quails, pheasants, and a variety of other birds. Deer are frequently seen crossing the trail in early morning or at dusk.

The trail is accessible from various crossroads and parking areas at designated spots, including Rochester, Rochester Hills, Oakland Township, Orion Township, and Lake Orion. To walk the stretch of the trail described here, park either at the lot on the north side of Tienken Road in Rochester Hills or the south side of Silverbell Road in Oakland Township.

Coming from Silverbell Road, you can pass the Tienken Road parking lot and follow the trail to a municipal park in downtown Rochester. Oakland makes for a nice starting point and adds a little more mileage to the trek if you walk all the way to the downtown park.

The trailhead off the Tienken Road parking lot is directly adjacent to the lot, on the east side. You'll see a large sign displaying a map of the linear trail, as well as a picnic table. From here, head left (north) along the trail.

The landscape from Tienken Road to Silverbell Road varies little but makes for an enjoyable scenic hike. For the most part, Paint Creek runs parallel to the trail on its western (left) shoulder. A thin tree line frames both sides of the trail, with impressive houses dotting either side. You'll cross the first bridge at about 500 feet. An expansive marsh stretches along the right side of the trail around the 0.5-mile mark.

Around the 1-mile mark, a short series of stairs on your right provides access to the creek. It's a nice spot to take pictures. About 0.1 mile later, you'll pass a small horse barn on your left. The trail crosses Dutton Road at the 1.2-mile mark; you'll spot a bench alongside the creek on your right.

As you approach the 2-mile mark, you'll see signs noting the remnant of a prairie on your right. The 1.2-acre prairie is home to various native species, including big bluestem and wild lupine. It's also part of a prairie restoration project. You'll reach Silverbell Road at the 2.2-mile mark. Turn around and retrace your steps to the starting point at Tienken Road.

Nearby Attractions

Walking less than a mile north on the trail from Silverbell Road, hikers will pass the Paint Creek and Goodison cider mills in the unincorporated village of Goodison. Tasty doughnuts and cider make both sites traditional autumn destinations. About 3.5 miles north, the trail abuts the Bald Mountain State Recreation Area, home to longer, scenic trails that traverse rolling terrain and thick woods.

Rochester boasts one of the most inviting downtowns in metropolitan Detroit. Boutiques, cafés, and restaurants, most of them independently owned, line Rochester Road, the town's main street.

The city's municipal park, which connects to the Paint Creek Trail, is just off Rochester Road. The downtown is home to well-attended festivals and art fairs. Among the noteworthy eateries is the Rochester Candy Shop at 436 S. Main St. The shop serves and sells a variety of Sanders products. Sanders, once an institution in metropolitan Detroit, is slowly making a comeback after nearly disappearing in the mid-1990s. The Rochester store sells the confectioner's rich ice-cream toppings, chocolates, and desserts.

Directions

From Detroit, take I-75 north to Rochester Road in Troy, Exit 67. Turn right onto Rochester Road and go about 9.5 miles to West Tienken Road. Turn left and go about 0.5 miles. The parking lot for the trailhead will be on your right, about 100 feet west of the intersection of Tienken Road and Kings Cove Drive.

From Ann Arbor, take US 23 to M-14 east. Follow M-14 to I-275 north, about 15 miles. Take I-275 to I-696 east. Go about 18 miles to I-75 north, Exit 18. Take Rochester Road, Exit 67. Turn right and follow Rochester Road about 9.5 miles to West Tienken Road. Turn left and go about 0.5 miles. The parking lot for the trailhead will be on your right, about 100 feet west of the intersection of Tienken Road and Kings Cove Drive.

Seven Ponds Nature Center Loops

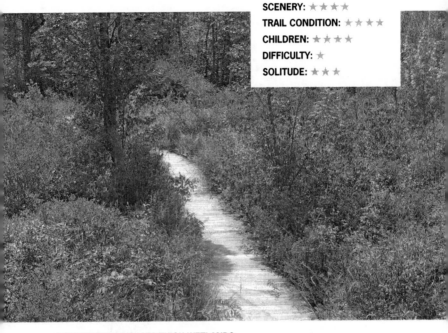

SCENERY: ★ ★ ★ ★
TRAIL CONDITION: ★ ★ ★ ★
CHILDREN: ★ ★ ★ ★
DIFFICULTY: ★
SOLITUDE: ★ ★ ★

A BOARDWALK BISECTS THICK WETLANDS.

GPS TRAILHEAD COORDINATES: N42° 55.640' W83° 11.339'

DISTANCE & CONFIGURATION: 2 miles of connecting loops

HIKING TIME: About 1 hour

HIGHLIGHTS: Small glacial lakes, wetlands, woods, reconstructed prairie

ELEVATION: 977 feet at trailhead, with no significant rise

ACCESS: Tuesday–Sunday, 9 a.m.–5 p.m.; members can access grounds sunrise–sunset; $3 adults; $1 children

MAPS: At the visitor center or **sevenponds.org**

FACILITIES: Visitor center, restrooms, picnic area

WHEELCHAIR ACCESS: None

COMMENTS: No pets allowed on trails.

CONTACTS: 810-796-3200; **sevenponds.org**

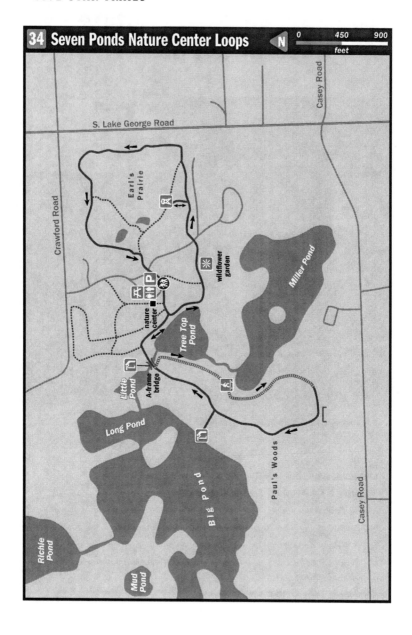

Overview

Dirt trails and boardwalks interweave around seven small lakes or ponds, formed by glaciers and connected by streams and channels. An A-frame bridge offers panoramic views of the ponds and wetlands and is a great spot from which to observe wildlife, including birds. A reconstructed prairie is home to native wildflowers; its observation deck offers an even broader view of the landscape. Summer and early fall are the best times to see the wildflowers.

Route Details

Several miles of trails crisscross the diverse landscape of the 468-acre Seven Ponds Nature Center near Metamora. This nature center is home to deep glacial lakes, ponds, marshes, fields, woods, and a reconstructed prairie. Trails dissect the entire property, some of them on an 80-acre section on the opposite side of Crawford Road known as the North-80. The trails connect to each other, and any number of combinations is possible. Sampling the loops between the ponds and around the prairie makes for an ideal hike and covers some of the center's most interesting terrain.

The most traveled trail is a loop that runs among five of the seven ponds, including two of the biggest, Big Pond and Miller Pond. Boardwalks, an A-frame bridge, and observation platforms bring hikers close to the wetlands and waterways, offering up close glimpses of aquatic life and waterfowl. It's common to see muskrats and beavers here, and more than 200 bird species have been sighted amid the woods and wetlands. Birders will be happy to know the latter includes nesting sandhill cranes, bluebirds, tree swallows, and swamp sparrows.

The trailhead is tucked amid a grove of pines just off the sidewalk at the southern edge of the visitor center. The trail slopes to lake level and a T-intersection. Straight ahead is a 40-foot-long dock extending into Tree Top Pond. Swing right, heading northwest, and pass a shed on your right. This short stretch is thick with trees. Tree

Top Pond will be on your left and the nature center is above, up the hill, on your right.

Swing left at the next intersection. This leads to the pond loop. The A-frame bridge, which overlooks Little Pond and Tree Top Pond, is directly in front of you. From there, the trail continues through marshlands and wet woodlands and reaches the next intersection at the 0.3-mile mark.

At the intersection, hikers may go left or straight to make the loop. Turning left heads to a boardwalk and Tree Top Pond. The long narrow boardwalk winds through marshland and along the edges of Tree Top Pond and Miller Pond before emerging in the woods. The Miller Pond boardwalk winds along the western shore of two ponds and cuts through a swamp forest; a platform overlooks an active beaver lodge. If you continue straight at the intersection, you'll follow the loop along Big Pond, but you will eventually wind your way back north along Miller and Tree Top ponds.

After following the Miller Pond boardwalk, the trail spills into the woods. Around the 0.6-mile mark, you'll cross an intersection. Swing right and follow the sign pointing the way to the nature center. To the left is a restricted access road. The stretch from this juncture and north to Big Pond is one of the most beautiful of the nature center trails, an area known as Paul's Woods. Sugar maples, oaks, hickory, and beech make up the mature forest. An occasional bench invites hikers to stop and take in the scenery. A spur on your left, near the 0.8-mile mark, leads to a wooden observation tower on Big Pond. It's the best spot for viewing ducks and geese.

Continuing northeast leads back to the A-frame bridge. Retrace your footsteps to the nature center, but instead of turning left at the dock, continue straight. The trail remains under a canopy of trees and passes by the Woodland Wildflower Garden, which features spring woodland flowers and ferns.

The trail reaches Earl's Prairie around the 1.3-mile mark and runs along the prairie's tree-lined edges. Your best bet is to bear right or straight at intersections to follow the outer loop around the perimeter of the 9-acre tract. Shortcuts dissect the loop, but they can be rather confusing. An observation tower stands at the loop's southern edge. Be sure to climb to the top for a panoramic view of the prairie and surrounding woodlands. Around 1.7 miles, you'll reach an intersection at the western edge of the prairie; bear right or straight, heading due west, crossing Crawford Road and arriving back at the visitor center.

Nearby Attractions

Four miles from the nature center is the Jonathan Woods Nature Preserve. The 145-acre tract is part of the nature center, and its varied terrain is home to mixed hardwoods, a beech-maple forest, a tamarack bog, yellow birch swamp, and a hemlock stand. It's an ideal place for observing wildlife and birds, including wood thrushes, scarlet tanagers, veeries, and waterthrushes. The woods also are home to barred owls and woodpeckers. There is no parking area; visitors should park at the preserve entrance.

Directions

From Detroit, take I-75 north to M-24 north, Exit 81. Drive M-24 about 19 miles. Turn right on West Dryden Road and continue for about 7 miles (it becomes West High Street and then East Dryden Road). Turn right on South Lake George Road and go 1 mile. Turn right onto Crawford Road. The nature center is on the left.

From Ann Arbor, take US 23 north to I-69, Exit 117A toward Flint-Port Huron. Follow the interstate about 22 miles and take Exit 155, M-24 toward Lapeer-Pontiac. Turn right onto M-24 and go about 6 miles. Turn left onto West Dryden Road and continue about 7 miles (it becomes West High Street and then East Dryden Road). Turn right onto South Lake George Road and go about 1 mile. Turn right onto Crawford Road. The nature center is on the left.

35 # Stony Creek Metropark:
East Lake Trails

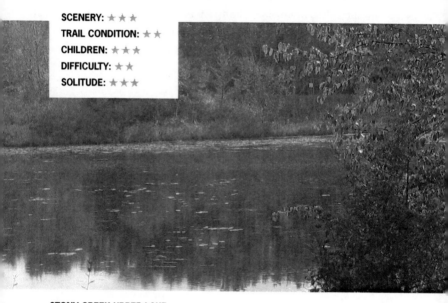

SCENERY: ★ ★ ★
TRAIL CONDITION: ★ ★
CHILDREN: ★ ★ ★
DIFFICULTY: ★ ★
SOLITUDE: ★ ★ ★

STONY CREEK UPPER LAKE

GPS TRAILHEAD COORDINATES: N42° 45.661' W83° 4.328'

DISTANCE & CONFIGURATION: 3.2-mile loop

HIKING TIME: About 1.5 hours

HIGHLIGHTS: Woodlands, fields, Stony Creek Lake

ELEVATION: 846 feet at trailhead, with no significant rise

ACCESS: May–October, daily, 6 a.m.–10 p.m.; November–April, daily, 7 a.m.–8 p.m.
Nature center: Monday–Friday, 1 p.m.–5 p.m.; Saturday–Sunday, 10 a.m.–5 p.m. $5 daily
fee; $25 annual pass

MAPS: At the nature center or **metroparks.com**

FACILITIES: Nature center, restrooms, picnic area

WHEELCHAIR ACCESS: None

COMMENTS: Bicycles and pets are not permitted on the trails. Picnicking in the nature
center area is allowed only at the picnic tables in the parking lot median.

CONTACTS: 586-781-9113; **metroparks.com**

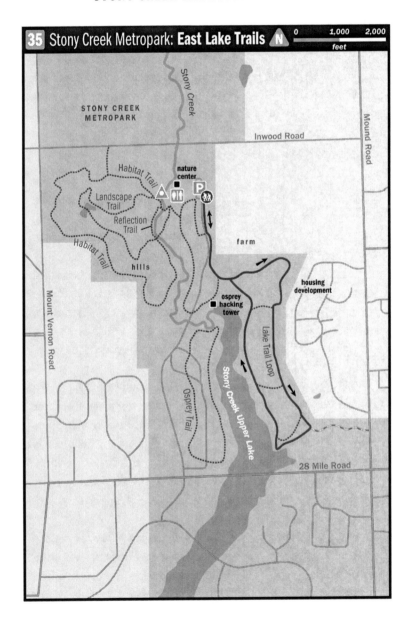

35 Stony Creek Metropark: **East Lake Trails** N

0   1,000   2,000

feet

STONY CREEK METROPARK

Inwood Road

Stony Creek

Mound Road

Habitat Trail

nature center

P

Landscape Trail

Reflection Trail

Habitat Trail

hills

farm

housing development

osprey hacking tower

Lake Trail Loop

Mount Vernon Road

Osprey Trail

Stony Creek Upper Lake

28 Mile Road

Overview

The East Lake Trails are a series of four connecting loops on the east side of Stony Creek Upper Lake. The trails are the most rustic of the Stony Creek Metropark Nature Center trails and wind mostly through woods and fields, and along the shores of Stony Creek Lake.

Route Details

Like its counterpart, Kensington Metropark in western Oakland County, Stony Creek Metropark is a favorite recreation destination. The 4,461 acres offer hiking, biking, fishing, golfing, picnicking, swimming, and wintertime sports of ice fishing, ice skating, sledding, and cross-country skiing.

Patterned after Kensington, Stony Creek Metropark opened in 1964. Its focal point—the lake—was created by damming Stony Creek, a tributary of the Clinton River. Thousands of years ago glaciers formed the creek, Reflection Pond, and the rolling landscape that today provide the park with one of the most varied landscapes of any of the metroparks.

There are plenty of choices for hiking at the metropark. The East Lake Trails are the most rustic of the nearly 9 miles of trails at Stony Creek Metropark Nature Center in the northeast section of the park. The southwest section has 14 miles of hiking and biking trails on the grounds of a former estate. Also a hit with bikers and walkers is an 8-mile paved trail that circles Stony Creek Lake. Lastly, 6 miles of trails are located in the Inwood section, at the far northern edge of the park.

Combined, the East Lake Trails are the longest of the five trails located at the nature center. Another trail in this area of the park is the 2.5-mile Habitat Trail, which winds through dense woods, wetlands, and broad fields southwest of the nature center. The 1.8-mile Osprey Trail loops along the western shore of Stony Creek Upper Lake and offers the best vantage point to see the osprey hacking tower.

The East Lake Trails begin at the southeastern edge of the nature center parking lot. Follow a wide grassy swath south as it runs parallel to the park road. At the first intersection, swing left, heading east and then due south. A sign marks the Lake Trail Loop.

From here, the trail winds in and out of the woods, through fields, and past a farm. As the trail loops around the eastern shore of Stony Creek Upper Lake, hikers will come across several intersections. These junctures create shorter loops, if you're inclined to cut distance. To follow the entirety of the outer loop, bear left at the next intersection and continue due east. The next intersection is less than 100 yards away on your right. Again, continue east, heading straight.

On its far eastern edge, the trail also cuts alongside a housing development before reaching another fork in the trail; this is one of two shortcuts along this stretch. Bear left, continuing south, through a field. The trail is a mix of woods and fields as its heads south.

Continuing along the full loop, heading south-southeast, hikers should also be aware of a confusing intersection when the trail turns westward toward the lake. The intersection is unmarked except for a sign noting a service drive. Swing right (west); if you continue straight, you're on the service drive heading to Mound Road.

The trail loops west and then runs north along the eastern shore of Stony Creek Upper Lake. A grassy area along a hill affords a panoramic view of the lake, the park, and even the bike path far on the opposite shore. The trail continues north, running parallel to the lake for a long stretch.

At the next fork, bear left through an open field; arrows help point the trail direction. The terrain becomes hilly and the trail narrows as it cuts deeper into the woods and along a ravine. Swing left at the next intersection and then right at the next. This leads back to the trailhead at the parking lot.

Nearby Attractions

North on M-53, Romeo is a well-known fall destination because of its ample apple orchards and cider mills. Among them are Hy's Cider Mill on 37 Mile Road, Stony Creek Orchard and Cider Mill on 32 Mile Road, and Westview Orchards on Van Dyke. The Inwood Trails north of the nature center are accessible by a spur off the Habitat Trail, and you may park on Inwood Road. The landscape features rolling fields, sparse woods, Inwood Lake, and ponds—ideal for a gentle walk and perfect terrain for cross-country skiers. But the trails are not as interesting as those in other areas of Stony Creek Metropark.

Directions

From Detroit, take I-75 north to Exit 67, Rochester Road. Turn right onto Rochester and drive 7 miles to Avon Road. Turn right and go 2 miles. Avon merges into Dequindre Road. Continue another 2 miles and turn right onto Mt. Vernon Road. Follow Mt. Vernon onto 26 Mile Road. The park entrance is about 1 mile farther on the right.

From Ann Arbor, take US 23 north to M-14 east. Follow M-14 about 15 miles to I-275 north. Go another 6 miles and merge onto I-696 east to Port Huron. Drive 18 miles to I-75 north, Exit 18, toward Flint. Follow that to Exit 67, Rochester Road. Turn right onto Rochester and go 7 miles to Avon Road. Turn right and go 2 miles. Avon merges into Dequindre Road. Continue another 2 miles and turn right onto Mt. Vernon Road. Follow Mt. Vernon onto 26 Mile Road. The park entrance is about 1 mile farther on the right.

Wolcott Mill Metropark:
Settler's Trail

SCENERY: ★ ★ ★
TRAIL CONDITION: ★ ★ ★
CHILDREN: ★ ★ ★
DIFFICULTY: ★
SOLITUDE: ★ ★ ★

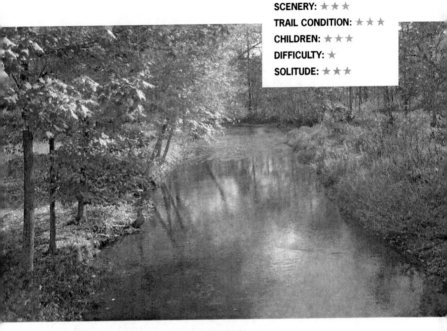

THE NORTH BRANCH OF THE CLINTON RIVER

GPS TRAILHEAD COORDINATES: N42° 45.934' W82° 55.727'

DISTANCE & CONFIGURATION: 1.9-mile loop

HIKING TIME: About 1 hour

HIGHLIGHTS: Woodlands, fields, northern branch of the Clinton River

ELEVATION: 659 feet at trailhead, with no significant rise

ACCESS: 9 a.m.–5 p.m., January–February, Friday–Sunday; March, Thursday–Sunday; April–December, Wednesday–Sunday; $5 daily fee; $25 annual fee

MAPS: At the gristmill at the historic center or **metroparks.com**

FACILITIES: Restrooms in the historic center, which includes the Wolcott Mill.

WHEELCHAIR ACCESS: Yes, at the historic mill, but not on the trails

COMMENTS: Leashes required for dogs and other pets. Bicycles prohibited.

CONTACTS: 586-749-5997; **metroparks.com**

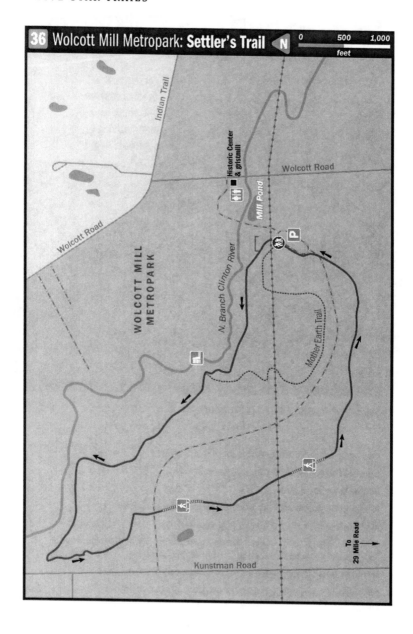

36 Wolcott Mill Metropark: **Settler's Trail**

Overview

Situated along the winding northern branch of the Clinton River, the historic Wolcott Mill looks like a slice of Americana that Norman Rockwell might have illustrated for the *Saturday Evening Post*. Towering maples and oak trees, flush in fiery colors in the fall, and green pastures help create one of the most pastoral settings in southeast Michigan. These mill grounds are the staging area for the park's most inviting trail, the Settler's Trail.

Route Details

The newest of the region's metroparks, Wolcott Mill is named after a gristmill that remains in the 2,625-acre park in northern Macomb County. Built in 1847, the mill was in continuous use by generations of the same family until 1967. Thousands of these mills once dotted Michigan's landscape, but today, only five remain in operation. Wolcott Mill, which displays grain-grinding machinery and other equipment, is an important reminder of the state's past.

The park is divided into four sections: the mill, Farm Learning Center, golf course, and Camp Rotary. The Settler's Trail and two smaller loops, the Mother Earth Trail and the Millrace Trail, are situated in the same area. The Settler's Trail is the most interesting of the three because it encompasses a broader swath of the park, meandering along the river and through fields and woods. The mill and other buildings are just a short walk away from the trailhead.

From the parking lot, head north-northwest, following a wide grassy path through a field to a large wooden sign marking the Settler's and Mother Earth trails. The trails are one and the same as you bear right, continuing to head in a north-northwest direction. The northern branch of the Clinton River will be on your right, just to the north. The Mother Earth Trail will eventually split from the Settler's Trail and continue its loop back to the trailhead. Instead, continue straight on the Settler's Trail. At about 130 feet, you'll reach a bench along the banks of the river. It's a perfect spot to take in the idyllic setting of the mill and the park. More river views can be seen along the trail.

The trail winds slightly away from the river, crossing through a field that becomes thicker with trees; most of the trees scattered near the beginning of the trail are new-growth trees. However, plenty of old-growth trees grow beside the route, especially along the river, thanks to the plantings of the property's original owner.

At a T-intersection, you'll see a sign with an arrow pointing the direction to the Wolcott Mill Dam; follow that guide, turning right, and continue north-northwest. The trail rises slightly, and you'll notice a magnificent beech tree growing from the side of a hill. A spur on your right leads to the concrete remnants of the dam, which helped control water to the mill. A storm in 1972 washed out the dam.

From here, the trail gradually rises higher and the river becomes harder to see as you walk under a thicker canopy of trees. Oaks, maples, black walnuts, and sycamores are common along the trail. The trail climbs 20–30 feet above the riverbanks, with steep slopes leading down to the flowing waterway. Around the 0.8-mile mark, a clearing offers another great view of the northern branch of the Clinton River. You'll hear water gurgling somewhere down below. The park's Farm Center, a 250-acre working farm with a herd of dairy cows, chickens, goats, pigs, horses, and sheep, is about 1 mile north, just up the river.

The trail bends west and turns in a southerly direction, crossing through a field with scattered trees. Around the 1-mile mark, you'll pass a grove of sugar maple trees, and you'll hear occasional cars and trucks entering and leaving the park entrance. Look for scattered white pines after the trail crosses the park entrance road and continues along a grassy pathway. The trail slopes gently and winds around a pond and along a boardwalk before crossing under power lines in a field. Around the 1.4-mile mark, the trail returns to the woods as it winds its way back to the park entrance road. The only notable break in the wooded landscape comes around 1.5 miles, when the trail crosses through a clearing. Trees and brush remain thick on either side, and you'll notice pines here and there. The trail eventually runs parallel to the park road. The trail ends just below the southern end of the parking lot, opposite of the trailhead.

Nearby Attractions

Wolcott Mill's working farm is an interesting diversion. The center's barn museum tells the history of American barns and displays antique farming equipment and a restored Model T dump truck. Twice a day April–October, and once a day the rest of the year, visitors can see the dairy herd being milked. The farm also grows a variety of crops, and the staff offers programs on subjects ranging from lamb and wool production to water conservation to modern farming techniques. The farm hosts frequent hayrides, and family programs take place at the Historic Center and Wolcott Mill throughout the year. The mill is open daily May–October and Wednesday–Sunday, November–April.

Directions

From Detroit, take I-94 east toward Port Huron for about 25 miles. Take Exit 241, 21 Mile Road. Turn left and go about 2 miles. Turn right on North Avenue. Go about 5 miles to 26 Mile Road. Turn left and go about 1.3 miles to Ray Center Road. Turn right. Follow the road north 3 miles to 29 Mile Road. Turn left and drive 2 miles to Kunstman Road. Turn right. The park entrance is less than 1 mile on the right.

From Ann Arbor, take US 23 north to M-14. Follow M-14 east about 15 miles toward Plymouth/Livonia. Merge onto I-275 north. Continue about 6 miles to I-696 east toward Port Huron. Go about 29 miles to I-94. Follow it east toward Port Huron. Take Exit 241, 21 Mile Road. Turn right onto North Avenue. Go about 5 miles to 26 Mile Road. Turn left and go about 1.3 miles to Ray Center Road. Turn right. Follow the road north 3 miles to 29 Mile Road. Turn left and drive 2 miles to Kunstman Road. Turn right. The park entrance is less than 1 mile on the right.

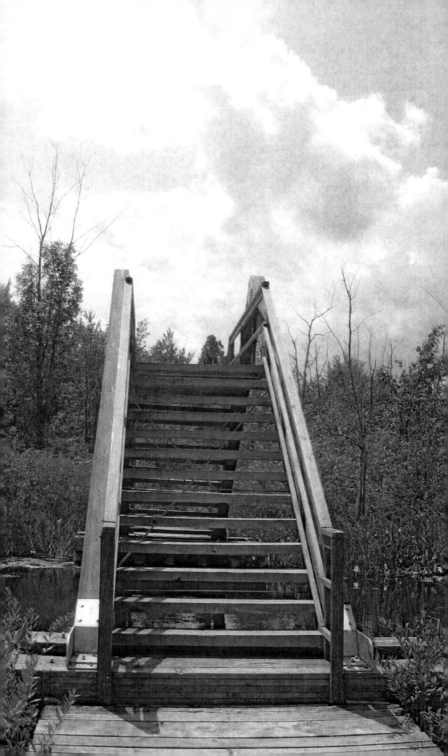

Appendixes
& Index

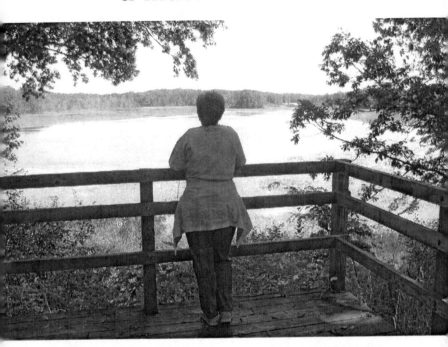

A HIKER ENJOYS THE VIEW OF WILDWING LAKE AT KENSINGTON METROPARK.

Appendix A: Outdoor Retailers

Following is contact information for outdoors retailers in the Ann Arbor and Detroit metro areas.

BASS PRO SHOP
basspro.com
Great Lakes Crossing
Auburn Hills, MI 48326
(248) 209-4200

BIVOUAC
bivouacannarbor.com
336 S. State St.
Ann Arbor, MI 48104
(734) 761-6207

CABELA'S
cabelas.com
110 Cabela Blvd. E.
Dundee, MI 48131
(734) 529-4700

DICK'S SPORTING GOODS
dickssportinggoods.com
9950 Village Place Blvd.
Brighton, MI 48116
(810) 225-4849

50580 Waterside Dr.
Chesterfield Township, MI 48051
(586) 949-0760

21061 Haggerty Rd.
Novi, MI 48375
(248) 735-8180

44225 12 Mile Rd.
Novi, MI 48337
(248) 596-3400

1290 S. Rochester Rd.
Rochester Hills, MI 48307
(248) 608-9696

23349 Eureka Rd.
Taylor, MI 48180
(734) 374-0429

400 John R Rd.
Troy, MI 48083
(248) 577-2879

45230 Northpointe Blvd.
Utica, MI 48315
(586) 254-2653

35500 Central City Pkwy.
Westland, MI 48185
(734) 523-0984

GANDER MOUNTAIN
gandermountain.com
43825 W. Oaks Dr.
Novi, MI 48377
(248) 380-4000

14100 Pardee Rd.
Taylor, MI 48180
(734) 287-7420

13975 Hall Rd.
Utica, MI 48315
(586) 247-9900

MOOSEJAW
moosejaw.com
327 S. Main St.
Ann Arbor, MI 48104
(734) 769-1590

34288 Woodward Ave.
Birmingham, MI 48009
(248) 203-7777

17370 Hall Rd. # 125
Clinton Township, MI 48038
(586) 416-8940

17037 Kercheval
Gross Pointe, MI 48230
(313) 881-9999

154 N. Adams
Rochester Hills, MI 48309
(248) 375-5800

THE NORTH FACE
thenorthface.com
2800 W. Big Beaver Rd.
Troy, MI 48084
(248) 816-2800

REI
rei.com
970 W. Eisenhower Pkwy.
Ann Arbor, MI 48103
(734) 827-1938

17559 Haggerty Rd.
Northville, MI 48168
(248) 347-2100

766 E. Big Beaver Rd.
Troy, MI 48083
(248) 689-4402

SPORTS AUTHORITY
sportsauthority.com
4220 Baldwin Rd.
Auburn Hills, MI 48326
(248) 333-1330

33930 S. Gratiot Ave.
Clinton Township, MI 48035
(586) 791-8400

5751 Mercury Dr.
Dearborn, MI 48126
(313) 336-6626

Appendix B: Places to Buy Maps

When you head out on hiking trails, the publisher and author strongly recommend that you carry other maps in addition to those provided in this book. Below are some good resources.

GARMIN
garmin.com

HURON-CLINTON METROPARKS
metroparks.com

REI
rei.com
970 W. Eisenhower Pkwy.
Ann Arbor, MI 48103
(734) 827-1938

17559 Haggerty Rd.
Northville, MI 48168
(248) 347-2100

766 E. Big Beaver Rd.
Troy, MI 48083
(248) 689-4402

TRAVEL MICHIGAN
michigan.org/things-to-do/outdoors/hiking/default.aspx

Appendix C: Hiking Clubs

The Ann Arbor and Detroit metro areas are home to many hiking enthusiasts. Here are some good contacts for clubs and groups that welcome your participation.

HIKING MICHIGAN
hikingmichigan.com

MICHIGAN ADVENTURERS CLUB
meetup.com/MI-adventurers

SIERRA CLUB CROSSROADS GROUP
sites.google.com/site/crossroadssierraclub

SIERRA CLUB HURON VALLEY GROUP
michigan.sierraclub.org/huron/index.asp
621 5th St.
Ann Arbor, MI 48103
(734) 668-6306

SIERRA CLUB SOUTHEAST MICHIGAN GROUP
michigan.sierraclub.org/semg/index.html
(248) 646-4113

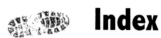

Index

About the Author

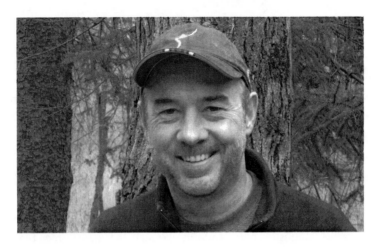

Northern Michigan was the first landscape **Greg Tasker** explored on foot. He began by following rural or abandoned roads through the woods around Oscoda and the Au Sable with his grandparents. Other times, hiking was simply a matter of exploring the rolling 80 acres of brush, thin woods, and pine trees at his family's Christmas tree farm near Cadillac. These were hikes without marked or maintained trails. He began hiking in earnest—on real trails—after moving to the East Coast, exploring famous and obscure trails from North Carolina to Vermont.

Tasker has written about hiking and outdoor activities for magazines that include *Scouting, Backpacker, AMC Outdoors, Vermont Life,* and *France Today*. His accounts have appeared in newspapers such as the *Baltimore Sun,* the *Pittsburgh Post-Gazette,* and the *Boston Herald.* As the Western Maryland correspondent for the *Baltimore Sun* in the mid-1990s, Tasker hiked extensively to write about the people and places of the state's mountainous region. Those stories included features on the Appalachian Trail, the C&O Canal Towpath, and others in the Maryland forests. As a travel blogger at the *Detroit News,* Tasker frequently writes about the trails and parks of southeastern Michigan.

DEAR CUSTOMERS AND FRIENDS,

SUPPORTING YOUR INTEREST IN OUTDOOR ADVENTURE, travel, and an active lifestyle is central to our operations, from the authors we choose to the locations we detail to the way we design our books. Menasha Ridge Press was incorporated in 1982 by a group of veteran outdoorsmen and professional outfitters. For many years now, we've specialized in creating books that benefit the outdoors enthusiast.

Almost immediately, Menasha Ridge Press earned a reputation for revolutionizing outdoors- and travel-guidebook publishing. For such activities as canoeing, kayaking, hiking, backpacking, and mountain biking, we established new standards of quality that transformed the whole genre, resulting in outdoor-recreation guides of great sophistication and solid content. Menasha Ridge continues to be outdoor publishing's greatest innovator.

The folks at Menasha Ridge Press are as at home on a white-water river or mountain trail as they are editing a manuscript. The books we build for you are the best they can be, because we're responding to your needs. Plus, we use and depend on them ourselves.

We look forward to seeing you on the river or the trail. If you'd like to contact us directly, join in at www.trekalong.com or visit us at www.menasharidge.com. We thank you for your interest in our books and the natural world around us all.

SAFE TRAVELS,

Bob Sehlinger

BOB SEHLINGER
PUBLISHER